"The very moment I met Jo, I knew she was one of God's finest treasures! Jo's unique ability to communicate the beauty of God's love has captivated me from our first conversation. She is able to explain the unexplainable, to accomplish the impossible, and to master the insurmountable! Soar Unafraid is one of the most compelling glimpses into the heart of God, through the unrelenting commitment of one woman. Never before have I cancelled an entire day in order to read a book!"

Erin Campbell
Executive Director/Producer
"Water through the Word" Broadcasting,
WaterThroughTheWord.com

"The title Soar Unafraid certainly fits this story; from Jo overcoming unbelievably painful feelings as she takes them to the Lord to chapters bubbling with joy and courage made possible by God. Throughout the book I see steadfast desire to live for and please God, and find a godly role model in Jo."

Jessica Shaver,
Author of *Gianna, Aborted and Lived to Tell About It*
and *Compelling Interests.*

SOAR
UNAFRAID
learning to trust no matter what

Anita,

Thanks for every thing!
my (you know I'm spacey!)
~~your~~ journey touch you

May in unexpected ways and

inspire you to...

Soar!
Love, Jo

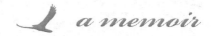 *a memoir*

SOAR
UNAFRAID
learning to trust no matter what

Jo Franz

TATE PUBLISHING & *Enterprises*

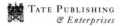

TATE PUBLISHING
& Enterprises

Tate Publishing is committed to excellence in the publishing industry. Our staff of highly trained professionals, including editors, graphic designers, and marketing personnel, work together to produce the very finest books available. The company reflects the philosophy established by the founders, based on Psalms 68:11,

"THE LORD GAVE THE WORD AND GREAT WAS THE COMPANY OF THOSE WHO PUBLISHED IT."

If you would like further information, please contact us:

1.888.361.9473 | www.tatepublishing.com

TATE PUBLISHING & *Enterprises*, LLC | 127 E. Trade Center Terrace

Mustang, Oklahoma 73064 USA

Soar Unafraid: Learning to Trust No Matter What

Book design copyright © 2007 by Tate Publishing, LLC. All rights reserved.
Cover design by Sarah Leis
Interior design by Jennifer Redden
Photography of Jo Franz by Bridget Belz

Published in the United States of America

ISBN: 978-1-6024709-2-7

1. Franz, Jo 2. Christian biography—United States 3. Autobiography—United States 4. Multiple sclerosis—United States—Biography 5. People with disabilities—United States—Biography 6. Divorce recovery—United States—Biography 7. Abuse—United States—Biography

07.04.11

To My Ray of Sonshine

Contents

Foreword

I met Jo when she was riding a tandem with her husband in the MS 150, a fundraising event for the National MS Society in Orange County, California, for which I served as vice president. She wore a sign on her back that read, "Thanks for Riding, I Have MS." My mom has MS and I was instantly drawn to Jo.

We grew to know each other, and I thought I knew what Jo had overcome in her life. But after reading *Soar Unafraid*, I felt I like I was getting to know another Jo, a Jo who had been through more than I had ever known. I am inspired by Jo's triumphs and her unwavering faith. She has had everything thrown at her to shake that faith, and she never falters. Her life is a testament to all those who are challenged with obstacles. Jo's deep faith, courage and perseverance are a lesson for all of us.

After finishing *Soar Unafraid* I couldn't get that sign out of my head— "Thanks for Riding, I Have MS." It's just like Jo. She faces the challenge and then shows gratitude to those around her. I am better for knowing Jo, and understand so much more after reading her story.

Katie Croskrey

Executive Director of the American Diabetes Association

San Diego, California

(Former vice president of the National MS Society in Orange County, California)

Preface

Ray and I descend in the elevator, after taking in the splendor of The Golden Room in Stockholm's City Hall. Decorated with 19 million fragments of gold leaf, the room hosts the annual banquet for the Nobel Prizes. Our tour group walks down the staircase as Ray takes me in a borrowed wheelchair into the Blue Hall. While our blonde guide says, "Thanks for being with us today," we look out through the courtyard windows to see fluffy snowflakes drifting slowly, then swirling wildly in a gust of wind.

"This should be fun!" I say with a grin as I tuck the blanket Inga gave me around my legs.

"At least we don't have far to go," Ray says.

He puts his gloves on and pushes me down the ramp into the courtyard, now covered in a white blanket of its own. Then he propels me through the crosswalk as cars slow down to wait for the man and woman caught in a spring snowstorm. We fly down the sidewalk of Norr Mälarstrand towards Inga's condominium and her waiting arms, ready for hugs and warmth.

"Stop, Baby! Take a picture of me right here all covered with snow. This is a memory we don't want to forget," I say, giggling.

Ray grabs our 35-millimeter camera, steps beneath a slight overhang, then clicks a shot we laugh over when we get our photos back on our return from Sweden.

Christer, another dear friend I made years ago, sends an e-mail we cherish—"It was wonderful to meet with you at Inga's place. It was such a long time ago. I also enjoyed talking to Ray—what a gift from God, when he gave you such a wonderful husband. I can see his love in his eyes when he looks at you."

I reminisce through the ups and downs of almost twenty years of marriage with Ray. We've been through so much together. And I can't help remembering what led up to this ...

Chapter 1

A Sure Diagnosis for an Unsure Me

"What's wrong, Jo?" Jenny says, grasping my arm as I wobble like a toy balloon body with sand in its bottom.

"I feel like I'm falling over."

I turn to see how the pancakes are cooking on the cast iron griddle and my head feels like it just keeps right on turning.

"Whoa," I say, as I land clumsily in the nearest chair, skidding across the speckled linoleum. "I've never felt so dizzy before."

By now, my husband, Ron, and the rest of his youth choir pours into our small kitchen to see what's happening. Burnt pancakes and sausage patties are smoking up the room as I say, "Get some fresh air in here, *please.*"

Ron obliges, exchanging concerned glances with Jenny while I try to laugh the whole thing off.

"Oh, well, there goes breakfast," I say, turning my attention to the hungry teenagers.

By the end of the long day I'm spent, like the toy balloon sprung a leak.

Several days later, standing at the kitchen sink I grab the counter to keep from falling over. I feel like a doll with its head on a spring, like the ones I've seen in the back window of cars. *What's wrong with me? Nothing,* I reprimand myself. *You always make a big deal out of nothing.* I remember falling down and hurting my knee in sixth grade ...

Dr. Purcell probes it here and there with his fingers, then says, "You're being a hypochondriac, Jo."

I *hate* that word—it means I am like my dad whose list of ailments annoys my mother. I sense her disdain whenever he expresses discomfort of any kind. My fear of being defined as a hypochondriac like him haunts me.

When I'm in my twenties Dad has triple bypass surgery. Mom shows compassion now, and when there are complications I notice worry lines deepening in her face, but between the crises, her impatience and annoyance with his problem seem to return.

Then she has her gallbladder removed and refuses to take medication though the long incision obviously hurts.

I ask, "What's wrong with dulling your pain for a day or two while your incision heals?"

Mom snaps, "I don't need it. That's why."

From the kitchen where I clean her refrigerator I hear her groaning as she moves about in my father's recliner, her body searching for a comfortable position. In my fear I can never measure up to her, I say, "Don't you *ever* clean this?" and immediately apologize. I'm criticizing her, hoping to elicit the very thing I hate to receive—guilt.

For months Ron and I pray God will heal me of the dizziness that bombards me like a buzzing fly at a picnic. Our prayer time excites us as we list prayer requests for friends, checking them off as God answers in some unique way or another. Our faith grows with every answered prayer, some of them miraculous.

As the bouts continue I grow increasingly frustrated because I *want* to believe God can heal me of this annoyance. I *want* to believe it's trivial, and I *don't* want to worry, but a nagging thought in the recesses of my mind will not let me rest. I wonder if I'm denying my belief in a faith that can move mountains when I say one spring evening, "I don't think I doubt God's ability to heal, but do you think I should see a doctor?" Ron agrees, and we write a new prayer request in our notebook—"Guide the doctor to diagnose the cause of the dizziness."

After a few tests I'm called in to see the internist for the results. I sit stiffly in the examining room on the aqua padded chair thinking, *there's nothing wrong with you. Face it. You're just like your dad.* The nagging thought still sits uneasily out of reach as the balding physician says, "There's nothing to worry about. Just an inner ear imbalance. If you start fainting, we'll prescribe something. Don't let it get you down."

So I decide I won't, even though unnatural fatigue zaps my strength. I fall asleep while Ron and I return from Cripple Creek with our friend Klas, who is visiting from Sweden. I *never* fall asleep in the car. I'm like a child on Christmas Eve when I'm in the Rockies. I love every vista. None of them looks the same to me, and every view entices me farther on around the next curve. But this time I snooze between red-haired Ron and blonde Klas in our Impala while I totally miss my beloved mountain scenery.

I have had trouble drifting off to sleep for as long as I can remember. A sense of angst, an anxiety I can't define, hits me the exact moment my head hits the pillow. I replay conversations of the day, hoping to understand what I could have, or should have, said differently. Then I list all that needs to be done the following day, week, or month.

My habit begins with *the nightmare* in early childhood. It seems to overwhelm me every single night. My heart pounds like a bass drum. I lay in a curled fetal position, terrified someone's coming towards my room. Sweat soaks the sheets as I shake uncontrollably. Floorboards creak louder as the person nears my door. But I can't scream for help. As hard as I try, no sound escapes my trembling lips. My mother suddenly appears at my bedside and rubs my back tenderly, saying, "It was just a nightmare, Jo, just a nightmare," as I sob fearfully.

I remember reading Nancy Drew mysteries as a young teen, hiding under my blanket with a flashlight. *Anything* but sleep. *The nightmare* ends sometime in high school, but it's as if giving in to sleep still isn't an option. By now I'm addicted. I have a gnawing need to stay alert when I lie down.

We take the doctor's advice to get on with life by packing our belongings for a move so Ron can begin seminary training. Several months ago, lying in bed, I said, "I think God wants us to do what we did in Stockholm last fall as our profession. You know how you've talked about enjoying our time there, telling people daily about our faith in God. I can't imagine doing anything else, can you?"

Ron said he'd been thinking about that, as well, and within a week he gave six month's notice at work.

Our boxes pile up as several of Ron's family members drive over to talk him out of this deviation from financial security which flies in the face of reason. Ron tells each relative one by one how important his faith is and how he wants it to be the driving force in his life. I beam with pride at his boldness for I know he's soft-spoken, rather shy most of the time, and he's struggled with confidence to lead the youth.

We move into a tiny, dark apartment after living in a "starter" house with a magnificent view of the Rockies. In the evenings I walk our basset hound, Jessie, after working for a radio news network. We traipse through fields of weeds that tangle her unusually long coat. I look furtively at the men hanging out in clusters at the edge of the field near their run-down houses. They're probably talking about their own day's work, but I can't help sensing their stares. I feel strangely frightened beneath them and wonder why. Relief floods over me once I'm behind locked doors.

Cockroaches skitter across the kitchen counter and a flash of anger surprises me. *I never had to deal with these vermin before.* Ron sits at his desk studying Greek. It suits him to learn the ancient languages of biblical times, and he seems oblivious to my unending battle to rid the apartment of the filthy cockroaches.

I'm a ninety mile-an-hour person trapped in a fifty-mile zone as naps consume my lunch hours so I can think in the afternoons. I used to decoupage, sketch, or paint during my evenings, even read a great book—always *busy,* multi-tasking, *doing* something rather than just sitting. Not any more. Within a couple months I can barely make dinner. Cooking and baking, simple loves, are now tiresome. The fatigue sits on my chest like a leaded dental x-ray shield. Tears come easily, more easily than ever before.

My hands and feet tingle and I have pain at the base of my skull. Much too often I have to call Ron to drive me home because I'm too dizzy. Frustration with my inner ear imbalance gives way to fear. I pray for God's strength to make it through the day because I'm reminded of a verse that says when I am weak, God will be strong (2 Corinthians 12:10). Then, amazingly, I have several symptom-free days, and wonder if I'm making them up. How can they come and go like this?

For the first time in years I remember a visit we made to my dad's parents in grade school. Every time we traveled to Grandpa and Grandma's I got sick, and this was no different. I sprawled on the upstairs poster bed and read the story of a little girl diagnosed with a fatal disease who is peaceful because she knows about God. I was moved to compassionate tears. Would *I* someday have a serious illness? I didn't tell anyone for fear I'd be humiliated for having such an absurd thought. As quickly as I entertained the horrifying prospect, I forgot it. I had to look happy. It's still the only way I feel loved and accepted. "Let's see that smile, Jo," my mom's mother says. I now wonder *could I be making myself ill?*

One day I walk down the hall at work and notice Roger leaning to his right as he walks towards me, so I ask why.

"Why are *you* leaning? I'm just mimicking you," he says. My eyes narrow with crinkled brows in disbelief. I don't even *know* I'm leaning to the left, mirroring Roger's fake list to the right. The nagging starts knocking again, but I block it out with escalating fear. *What's wrong with me, God?*

It's Christmas and we've been gone five months. With the money Ron's parents give us he buys gifts intended to relieve some of my fatigue—a vanity chair and lighted mirror so I can sit as I apply my makeup. His letter to me is full of devotion and gratitude for what I mean to him. Any woman would yearn for such a gift. I feel appreciated and loved. *Somehow,* I say to myself, *after eight years of marriage we'll weather this escalating storm together.*

I remember seeing the unexpected hurt on my mother's face as I answered her friend's question, "Are you looking forward to your move?" with my enthusiastic, "*Yes.*" Mom acted personally insulted. I'd been thrilled about the adventure of our new life, but now it's our first Christmas away and we miss our families. We play John Denver's *Rocky Mountain High* album as we turn on the gas fireplace.

After returning home from our friends' villa the phone rings and Ron hands it to me, mouthing—it's your mother.

"Merry Christmas! So, how was your day?" she asks a little too cheerfully, with a hint of something else. I answer, "We had a good time. Spent it at friends'. Only problem was my dizziness. I leaned, bumping into tables and hanging onto walls. I nearly knocked over a chair!"

"Oh, come on now, Jo. If you'd just think more positively, you wouldn't be so dizzy," Mom says. When I quickly end the call Ron tells me I look like I've been slapped. His freckles fade under his reddening face showing just how furious he is. My inability to measure up to Mom's standards soars to new heights as my equilibrium plummets to a new low. *How could I make this up?* I wonder as I crumple on the bed.

I lie here replaying our brief conversation. I told her I didn't feel like talking further when tears began to flow. I bury my face in my pillow and cry softly, so as not to wake Ron. *I shouldn't be surprised at Mom's response.* I've been praying for God to help me battle the criticalness I grew up with—subtle nitpicking frequently giving way to cutting remarks— "Why can't you do anything right?" "Oh, get out of the way, let me do it." And how we pestered and made one another the butt of our jokes. I remember a girlfriend playing with me when my brother, Doug, came into the room and began teasing me. When I got upset he called me "prune face" and my friend joined in, mocking me. I wanted to relax and "take a joke," but didn't know how to laugh at myself. So I stuffed my emotions deep inside myself, fearing their laughter would grow so loud Mom would come in and join them by saying, "Come off it, Jo, you always blow things out of proportion. Grow up."

When I succeeded in denying things hurt me, I put on the mask of cool indifference. But when I couldn't, I either spoke defensively or cried uncontrollably, all the while telling myself how stupid I was. The torrent of tears I tried to hold in exploded, and I felt guilty for having cried on top of the pain of having feelings in the first place, and then I would tell myself I was *bad*. I feel bad *once again*.

Over the next few weeks various specialists rule out possible causes for my symptoms. Every negative test result leaves me more anxious. My mouth feels dry as a desert, yet my palms moist as I wait in the sterile white hospital room for Dr. Black, my neurologist. Can he feel my racing pulse as he reaches his hand out to shake mine? *Don't be afraid.* I *will* myself to believe God is with me. Dr. Black probes my left side with a needle. It feels *numb*. My right side tests weaker than the left. *That's* why I lean to the left as I walk. I nearly kick Dr. Black as he gently taps below each of my kneecaps. Fear shoots through me, shattering the peace I try to claim. Dr. Black suggests a tiny, operable brain tumor the size of a pea could cause all of my symptoms. I want to sigh with relief, but he suggests it could also be something called demyelinating disease. That same nagging thought chokes back any relaxed breaths I might allow myself.

As Dr. Black leaves I look around feeling lost. I'm glad I don't have a roommate—some stranger staring at me—the one who believes in God, but who doesn't know where to turn at the moment. *Ron's teaching a guitar lesson, I shouldn't disturb him.* I dial our pastor's number.

"Hi, this is Jo. I was wondering if I could talk to you for just a minute. My neurologist was just here and he said—"

"We're having dinner. I'll have to call you back," he says abruptly.

"Oh. Sure. That's fine," I say, embarrassed for interrupting him, though I thought it was long after the dinner hour. *I know pastors need their private time, what am I doing?* He doesn't call later, but I don't notice that evening.

Next, I call Marsha. She and Jeff moved here in the same U-Haul truck with Ron and me—two young couples leaving home for the chance to serve God by serving others.

"Marsha, I hope I'm not bothering you," I say and she answers, "Not at all, Jo, how *are* you?"

"Well, the neurologist was just here. He said I might have an operable brain tumor. Or something called demyelinating disease."

Marsha cries, "Oh, Jo, would you like me to come to the hospital to be with you?"

Tears escape my eyes at the sound of her concern. "No thanks. Visiting hours are over. It helps just to talk with you. To know you care," and I begin to cry. "Ronnie will be finished with his lesson soon and I can talk with him. Thanks so much."

I dial our home as soon as Marsha and I hang up, and Ron asks, "Hi, honey, what did the neurologist say?" After I explain I hear a pregnant silence before he asks, "Is demyelinating disease serious?"

"I don't know. I didn't ask," I say. "I called Pastor Bill to talk to him, but he was busy, so I called Marsha. I didn't want to interrupt your lesson."

Again, I hear silence before Ron says with hurt in his voice, "You could've called me." I sniff and say, "I'm sorry. I love you." Ron replies, "Ditto," with a softer voice. "I'll see you tomorrow."

I'm sitting up in bed crying, feeling terrible for hurting Ron, wondering why I didn't call him in the first place, when the night shift nurse comes in to check on me.

"You okay, sweetie?" she asks and I answer, "Sure," dabbing my eyes. "Sure," I repeat again as I cry out inside, *God, help me!*

In the morning I lie perfectly still for the spinal tap. I'm told to keep my head down and I do, but within minutes it throbs. When my neurologist tells me I have a spinal headache, I defend myself, "But, I kept my head down, I haven't lifted it *at all.*"

Dr. Black says, "It's not your fault. This happens to some people when the needle hole doesn't seal right away. Your spinal fluid is leaking into your back. We'll give you something for the pain and keep you lying flat. It will eventually close on its own and the spinal fluid will cushion your brain again."

My once small waist fills with spinal fluid. I look like a thick tube days later when an anesthesiologist injects some of my own blood into my back to form a huge bruise to close the hole. I keep thinking I must be doing something to increase the problem though my kind nurses deny it.

Ron does his homework in my room after we've eaten together, and tonight he tells me, "Jessie misses you." I miss her, too. I miss her huge front paws landing on me with her hello even though I've become so weak she could easily knock me off balance. My constant headache overwhelms me this evening. It's lasted ten days. I can't hold in the tears. Ron scoots his chair close to the right side of my bed, and he begins singing a duet from our concerts. I harmonize softly along with him. It's a song about asking God to part the waters when I feel like I'm drowning.

"Thank you, Ronnie," I say through my tears as he squeezes my hand and kisses me.

When Dr. Black pushes open the door in the morning, he enters a room transformed by loving concern and compassion. Cards from dear friends, acquaintances, and even strangers, who've heard about me at seminary, cover the radiator underneath the wall-length window and line the shelf above the suspended television. Colorful arrangements of all kinds of cheerful flowers brighten the inherent drabness of the room. My worn Bible lies on my food tray. Ron sits in the tan vinyl chair he's claimed near the window, a theology book open on his lap.

"Jo," Dr. Black says after a warm hello to both of us, "Your test results indicate demyelinating disease. Another name is multiple sclerosis."

I *should* feel like a bomb has dropped on us, exploding into fragments of lost hope, but the now familiar thought announces itself as Ron says, "We thought it might be that."

"*Really*, why's that?" Dr. Black says.

"Because we have a friend who has MS," I say. "And because of her I went door-to-door raising funds for the National Multiple Sclerosis Society a year ago, so we know quite a bit about it. I was afraid you might think I was a hypochondriac if I diagnosed myself, so I didn't say anything." *Not that I want to have MS. I've denied it for months.*

Dr. Black smiles as he scribbles a note. "You're very intelligent. I think you'll do just fine. I suggest you look up a neurological textbook at the medical library that I'm writing down for you, Ron, and make copies of the pages about MS. If you can accept what *might* happen, you'll be prepared for whatever does. I hope you have a very benign course with the disease." He hands Ron the piece of paper, saying, "Jo, we need to get your headache under control before I can release you. If you fall you'll endanger your brain without the spinal fluid protecting it. We'll continue treating your MS with steroids. While you're here you can read through those pages and ask me any questions you come up with."

After he leaves, Ron and I calmly discuss options. Our desire to give concerts, like we have a number of times, with one-night stands traveling in a motor home sounds too tiresome. And ministry overseas might not be covered by our insurance. We talk as though we have taken the wrong turn on a road, but no problem, here's another route; we can still get there from here. We aren't terrified. We aren't angry. It isn't until months later that I learn Ron cried while sharing the news during a long distance call to the husband of our friend with MS.

After Ron leaves I actually feel relieved to have a diagnosis for symptoms my family seems to think I'm making up. Strange that I would be glad to *have* an illness rather than have imaginary symptoms. Tears trickle onto my pillow. My thoughts traverse valleys of fear, raging torrents of uncertainty, and mountains of impending challenges. I *know* what MS can do. I can develop GI, bladder or bowel problems; become blind, weakened, numb, or even paralyzed. There are no *human* cures for MS. There are no proven treatments. Only steroids to slow down an MS attack and hopefully cause less disability.

A note I received begs the question on my mind—"You've just committed to serve God with your life. Why has he allowed this to happen *now?* I don't understand." *I don't understand either, God. How can I serve you when I have MS? I'll need so much more energy than I have. Why now, when we've just begun seminary? At least I know you love me. I haven't always known that.* I think back …

My buddies from the band must've jumped in Dan's Malibu right after my distress call, because they honk within twenty minutes. I run out of my folks' house, slamming the heavy front door on my way to the Chevy.

"Thanks, guys. You're the best," I say, blowing air through my mouth with a protruding lower lip in sync with the door closing. "I just want to get drunk. My dad's been laid off *again* and my parents are arguing! If there *is* a God, he must have forgotten where my family lives! My parents go to church and give money every Sunday. How can God treat them like this?"

By now I'm shouting and hot tears soak my mascara so it runs in black rivulets down my face. Not only are my friends shocked by my outburst, I am too. I usually cloak my feelings in a giddy façade with friends. But I look at my parents' marriage as a piece of Mom's fine crystal, getting chipped with each argument, and somehow I must be to blame for its shattering. I'll do anything to mend my parents' palpable silence after they yell at each other. When they glower, seething in anger, speak in sarcastic tones, or swear, I feel like an utter failure. Like tonight—I just can't take it tonight.

Getting ready to enter my sophomore year of college, I wonder if things will ever change at home. I live in terror when Dad drives angrily, speeding, yelling profanities at other drivers while careening past them dangerously. I try to make excuses for his frequent sales job changes, just as I strive to give Mom compassion when he sulks over dinner, and I realize she'll never receive praise for even one tiny pay-raise. Mom stays in the same position until she retires, afraid of risking the only job security our family has.

I anesthetize myself with alcohol this summer night like I have at parties since ninth grade. I mask dejection and inner turmoil with party-girl cheerfulness, at times drinking until I don't know where I am or who I'm with, trading kisses for drags from guys' cigarettes until I decide my singing career could be destroyed by a raspy smoker's voice, and I quit taking even an occasional puff.

The thrill of my life is singing with these friends in our folk/soft rock band. When I'm singing I actually *feel* happy, I don't have to *act* happy, like when Grandmother sees me crying or sad and tells me to go into the bathroom and wash my face and put on a smile before I come back out. During the week I study on a classical voice scholarship at the University of Colorado. On weekends I wear a short psychedelic striped dress and serenade crowds in smoky clubs with my favorite solo. The haunting "Both Sides Now"[1] describes my life perfectly—I don't understand *any* of it—in and out of relationships, looking for some kind of meaning, some kind of love.

Thanksgiving Eve of 1972. Ron and I've been married three years. As we sit among thousands of others waiting for The 5th Dimension's concert to begin in a huge auditorium, I catch the eye of the woman seated on my right. Her nose crinkles in the cutest way when she smiles. Our conversation flows freely to personal information I don't expect. She and her husband reiterate how their faith in God makes all the difference when life is difficult.

I'm caught totally off guard when Judie Rice asks if I am a Christian. *That's for church, not here. Not at a concert.* Meanwhile, my brain, like a computer, instantly displays this data on the monitor screen of my mind—taken to *Christian* church services as a child, not another world religion. So, with confidence I say, "Yes, I'm a Christian." It doesn't matter that I doubt God really cares *if* he even exists.

Now Judie asks, "Do you know Jesus in a *personal* way?" My face contorts in confusion as I say, "How do you do that?" Judie smiles broadly as she pulls a booklet out of her purse and begins to read it. I stare at this couple and wonder—*if I'm a Christian, why don't I believe in God the way Judie and Marshall do? Except for my Grandmother, who can't help talking about God as if he's real, the Christianity I've experienced seems hypocritical. That's why I quit attending church years ago, besides maybe Christmas and Easter.*

I'm relieved when Randy Newman enters the stage for his warm-up act, immediately joking about how small he is. I don't have to think about the enormity of what I've just heard—that Jesus died for *me*—because no matter how hard I try, I can't be good enough for God. And I need to believe he sent his Son, Jesus, to die in my place in order to *experience* God's love. Regardless of how much I want to get lost in some of my favorite 5th Dimension songs of all time, "Up, Up, and Away" and "Grazing in the Grass," I can't totally block out the sparkle I see in Judie and Marshall—

I've never seen that in anyone before. I feel empty. Earlier this very evening, as I sat across from Ron in a romantic Italian restaurant, the title line from the popular song "Is That All There Is?" played over and over in my mind like a scratched record. I never really thought about it before tonight, but I *do* want something more in life.

As we leave the auditorium arena and walk out into the chilly air, exuberant men and women scatter across the crowded sidewalk handing out flyers about Jesus, of all people. I've never encountered these Jesus Freaks before, though I've seen them on the news. "Jesus Loves Me" plays in my head now. I learned it in Sunday school. But the Jesus I heard about did not care about me *personally,* he cared about *every*body. *Is someone trying to tell me something?*

During the drive home I think about my life, and realize everything I have—my husband, house, job, dog, hopes of children—could be gone in an instant, and what would I live for? Nothing. I feel even more hopeless about life's meaning. When I walk into our house from the garage, I barely notice Jessie's playful "Rrrrfff" for attention, because I can hardly wait to devour the booklet Judie gave me. For the first time in my life I realize that going to church does not automatically make me a Christian. I realize I can't use the way other Christian people live, or don't live, as a cop-out. I'm responsible for myself. I've always thought I was a good person—I don't cheat on my income taxes, I take change back to clerks who give me back too much, I care about my neighbors. But for the first time ever, because the booklet quotes a Bible verse that says, "All have sinned and fall short of the glory of God" (Romans 3:23), I realize even a snotty remark takes me out of God's category. I've hated the word "sinner." Now I realize I am one.

I kneel beside my bed. I don't know why I kneel, I just do, asking God's forgiveness for my desire to live my life apart from him, for my sin. I don't see visions or hear bells, but I feel loved like never before. It's as if God says, *"You are worth more than anything in the world to me,"* and I can't comprehend a love that vast. The booklet says God has a plan for my life. What will God have in store for me now that I've become his child? God *is* real. He knows where I live and he *cares* about me. I eagerly give my life to him, not knowing what that really means, hoping he'll fill the emptiness with his love and a purpose for living.

I lie in my hospital bed remembering the evening I came to know Jesus loved me over five years ago. If God had laid out then the plan for my life, I might have run the other way as fast as I could. Yet God wouldn't send his Son, Jesus, to die for me only to withdraw his love later on. He wouldn't waste that incredibly painful sacrifice by turning his back on me when I'm ill. *Thank you for reminding me of your love for me. No matter what happens with MS, Lord, I've got to remember I can trust you somehow.* Tears of another kind, a gratitude welling up within me, now wet my pillow.

Looking over at cards on the windowsill, my gaze falls on one whose message puzzles me. A close friend wrote—"God must think you're very special. He knows how you'll handle this." *I don't even know how I'll handle MS. How can she possibly think that? How do you want me to handle it, God?* Two sisters from church visited yesterday, and we laughed as I joked about my steroid-filled chipmunk-cheeks. *I'm trying to live out the verses that say be joyful. Does being able to laugh about something mean I'm joyful, God?* I'm not usually funny. That doesn't seem to be what the verses mean. I heard from another friend today that when the Laughlin sisters left here they felt *I* encouraged them more than they encouraged me. *Does that prove I'm joyful?* I learned something years ago I need to remember ...

Three years after becoming a Christian, we're moving Grandmother. As Ron and my brother lug Grandmother's couch through the doorway, the hide-a-bed begins to open up and I reach to close it, only to be pinned in between the door jam and the bed trying to reveal itself. Later, sharp pains stab my chest with every breath I take.

"Costochondritis," the doctor says, "torn cartilage in the chest. You need to see a physical therapist (PT) for ultra-sound treatments."

And so my PT visits begin.

For days I struggle to believe *my* inconsequential health problem is worthy of God's attention. Then I read how much Jesus cares about *every* need. Just as I'm about to ask God to heal the Costochondritis so I can sing for him, I remember how the Bible explains that when we praise God during difficult times, our focus evolves from what we *want* to have changed to what God can do in our lives in the *midst* of our problem. Our praise is a sacrifice of what we want or think we need, as Hebrews 13:15 explains, "Through Jesus, therefore, let us continually offer to God a sacrifice of praise—the fruit of lips that confess his name." So, I kneel beside my bed, gingerly lean on my arms and pray, "I praise you because you are God. I'm so glad you love me."

Though I'm not sure this is good theology, I open my Bible randomly. Verses in Hosea 6 say that though God has torn, he will heal. He will revive after two days and restore on the third day. It says keep trying to know God and he will come to me like spring rain. I look up wide-eyed to hear rain splatter in huge drops against the windowpane. More words of praise pour from my mouth.

On the second day since I praised God, after a few weeks of ultrasound treatments, my pain subsides tremendously. On the third day it stops *altogether*. I feel a sense of wonder I can't describe as I decide I want to learn to praise God at all times. When I tell my PT my pain has disappeared, I discover she sincerely listened as I looked up into her face during each appointment and told her about my relationship with Jesus. Sherri became a *Christian!* The happiness I feel at Sherri's news makes the Costochondritis worthwhile. It hasn't gone to waste. I would probably *never* have met Sherri if I hadn't needed physical therapy.

As I lie in my hospital room I flip through Bible pages, reading in 1 Thessalonians 5:18 that I'm to live joyfully, pray constantly, and give thanks no matter what's happening in my life because it's God's will. *You know I pray continually, I praise you now more than ever, and I'm thankful for your love. Is that what it means to be thankful in all circumstances? You don't really mean for me to be thankful for MS, do you? Am I to be thankful like I was with the Costochondritis? I don't know how to be joyful in this, but I want to learn. Help me, please, God.* Tears of exhaustion and blinding pain escape my eyes while

I hear every squeaking chair at the nurses' station, every sound of footfalls down the hall, every cough on my floor. I ring the bell fastened to my sheet and request some relief for my sleeplessness.

The stiffly starched nurse's cap appears before the scowling woman's face. "You need to accept your diagnosis, young lady!" she says.

"I'm trying. Doesn't that take some time?"

"I see you have a Bible open," she says, pointing, her finger dripping with conviction. "God cannot be pleased with you!" *This nurse doesn't know how much I want to trust you, God!* I cry as she stalks out of my room. I lay awake most of the night thinking about the life of Joni Eareckson, whose autobiography[2] Klas gave me before he left last summer. She riled at God about the quadriplegia after her diving accident, but then she gradually learned to accept that God had a plan for her in the wheelchair. "God, I pray you'll heal me totally of MS, but if not, help me to live like Joni does, relying on you."

Chapter 2

New Life with MS Haunted by the Old

I can't read the neurology pages during my twenty-eight day hospital stay—my brain is fuzzed by pain killers and steroids. I already know multiple sclerosis means "many scars," and the fatty tissue protecting the nerves, called myelin, is lost leaving scar tissue known as plaques or lesions. The central nervous system (CNS) is attacked by an autoimmune response and when myelin or nerve fiber is destroyed or damaged, the nerves ability to conduct electrical impulses is disrupted, producing various symptoms. At home I read more than I want to know. Ron looks at it and we don't act afraid to each other, but alone I'm frightened as I wonder if MS will affect me like it did the photographed severely disabled woman. What will my husband think if I become like that?

In order to accept what's happening, I begin journaling ongoing symptoms. Within a month I notice an intermittent burning sensation in my legs, feet and arms; patchy goose-bumps; recurrent blurred vision; weakness in my arms and legs; and scattered numbness. When I lower my head, an electrical sensation shoots down my torso and legs; and my ears deafen, only to ring out until I can hear again. I hope my MS diary will help. We've decided to enroll me in a cancer and MS research program utilizing injections formulated from a factor of donors' white blood cells.

Hoping I've experienced my only bad spell and will remain in remission, I return to work. Then Ron and I spend hours at an amusement park, and the next day I'm hanging onto walls as if on a boat being rocked at sea, while carrying a bag of heavy laundry. Dr. Black puts me back on steroids, which I hate. They hype me up so I have even more difficulty sleeping. My skin crawls. My mouth and stomach feel raw. I must reduce working to half-days due to lingering daily fatigue. Once I reach this exhaustion level, I think through a fog and my body feels limp.

Letters arrive from friends in Sweden, with Klas writing though he's sad—"I understand you love each other and trust in the Lord more than ever." Christer, the youth director of the church, Kirka vid Brommaplan, writes—"I was very shocked ... I am thankful to the Lord he has given you power to praise him in this hard situation, and for me and the youth in the church it is a strong witness."

My girlfriend since fifth grade says in her letter—"I praise him for your beautiful acceptance in faith ... I'm marveling at God ... the way he has prepared you both in spiritual maturity and knowledge of his loving concern and plan for your lives. Much love, Carolyn."

Ron and I are relaxing for a change when we hear a barely audible knock. Ron invites in the young man from a local church, and as we chat, MS comes up. He says, "I'd like to pray for you, if that's okay," and I say, "Sure."

As he prays for me to be totally healed of MS I'm agreeing silently, *yes, this is what I want.* Then he says, "Give this lady more faith to *claim* your healing. More faith than she's *ever* had before." Ron and I thank him and say good night.

"Ronnie, I want my faith to be growing all the time, but how can I ever make sure I have *enough* faith to be healed? Who, but Jesus, says what's enough?"

Ron shakes his head as if to emphasize his, "I don't know."

The prayer only magnifies my struggle. I've prayed fervently for healing with every ounce of faith I can muster. I've searched through the Bible to understand the "more faith" outlook. A father, pleading with Jesus to heal his son, *if he could,* asked Jesus to help him with his unbelief (Mark 9:23–24). I'm praying that, too. Can I *claim* healing when God's answer to the apostle Paul's request was "No" (2 Corinthians 12:8–9)? How can I be sure it's God's will to heal *me?*

Just before we move to where Ron will direct a youth program while continuing studies, we're asked to share at a party for seminary students and their wives. As Ron accompanies us on his acoustic Martin guitar, I weave solo lines into harmonies with his tenor voice. Our songs are laced with hope I feel at this moment, as if a filigree web holds us from the path of uncertainty lying ahead.

I say, "Admittedly, we're just learning how to give thanks in all circumstances and for all things. We'll have challenges with MS." Ron nods. "But none of us has guarantees." I pause, as if taking them to a door marked— Unpredictable Life Ahead, Proceed with Faith. "I want to replace what I may no longer be able to do with something I can, not focus on losses. Please pray this is the life we lead, bringing glory and honor to God. Thank you," and my throat chokes on an expanding lump as Ron squeezes my shoulder.

I'm excited to help people as a pastor's wife, but I don't know how much I can do with MS. I fight giants of guilt who shout down, "You should accomplish more!" I'm as dependent upon worry as a person who needs tobacco, alcohol or drugs. Even as I pray to give up my addiction, I notice I'm not trusting God with fears, only amplifying my guilt, keeping me in an imaginary gerbil's cage—running round and round with anxiety—triggering a sense of being *bad* for feeling it, which I confess and ask forgiveness for, but can't always accept. This propels me into guilt that I'm a Christian who feels *too good* for God's forgiveness. And the wheel keeps turning. Without knowing why I'm like this, worry is my sense of control when I feel out of control. All the while I want to stop worrying because I know *God's* in control. On occasions when I sense I *am* forgiven, the wheel screeches to a stop, and God's unconditional love floods me with a peace I can hardly bear, it's so diametrically opposed to my upbringing.

My plea becomes, "I *want* to trust you, God. Cause me to relax and be happy so Ron isn't disappointed in who I'm becoming because of MS." And I pray almost daily, "Give me compassion, and bridle my short tongue. I blow it so often."

One day I walk into Ron's office and sit in the wingback chair facing him. I say, "Ronnie, wouldn't it be great if we could get more youth to attend the Sunday evening class you're teaching? Kids get bored so easily. Why don't you think of ways to make it more exciting? You're doing a great job, but—" I say, not thinking how it comes across. Ron's face falls.

"I'm sorry. I didn't mean for it to sound like that. It's not your teaching. The material's dry. I'm bringing it up because *you're* discouraged about attendance." *What have I done?* "Ronnie, I'm so sorry," I cry, knowing I've just blasted his fragile confidence. "Is there any way I can help?"

Ron looks down, swallows, and tilts his head. He's trying to recover from the criticism, trying to accept my apology. He says, "I think it would be good if you'd make some visual aids, but I need to do this."

He buries his head in a theological book and I know the conversation is over. I hate it when I've hurt him or someone else and don't feel forgiven. It's as if I've been set out to sea in a boat without sail or motor. I don't know how to *fix* it, to heal the breach. I fear I'm banned forever from the presence of the one I wounded needlessly. Fear threatens to punch holes in the boat, sinking me to the depth of the sea. Crying out to God for forgiveness, I seek fresh wisdom for a solution to the hurt I've inflicted, the aloneness I feel.

I back out of the room feeling terrible, especially when my heart's desire was to help. I chastise myself for not thinking through what I wanted to communicate before speaking. Even though Ron's told me my zeal for God is frequently an impetus for his own growth, I've sounded judgmental.

So often when I want to encourage someone I immediately apologize, only to be told, "That's okay. I know what you mean" or "I didn't take it that way at all. Thanks for telling me." I feel like wearing an internal muzzle so I don't sound critical. I journal— "God, I've prayed for *years* for you to change this in me. When will I learn? Please help."

It's June and I relish being involved in every activity, but afterwards the only way I can get around is to crawl. MS hounds me like a starved coyote. Did I push too hard? Ron wanted me with him. Grandmother writes— "Jo, this is a scolding! I can't think God is pleased for you to forget your health, the body is the temple of the Lord. Now Darling, we all love you so much." I'm frustrated. When I admitted to feeling dizzy I heard—be positive. When I go on with life and downplay MS—I'm selfish and ungodly. My family's lack of approval hangs over me like thunderclouds. I've been under them before.

Mom begins working when I turn seven, and by eight I'm cooking most dinners during the week— "a little mom." I especially like making desserts for Dad, and when he praises me I beam. But if he says, "Now, let's get hot fudge sundaes!" my tiny heart breaks—my attempt obviously wasn't satisfying enough. I put on a grin so as not to hear, "Jo, you're too sensitive!"

I also want Mom to be proud of me. One day Dad takes me to her office. Her fellow employee says, "You're such a sweet girl, Jo." I hear Mom snort, like she disagrees. Why would Mom mind someone complimenting her daughter?

One Saturday I lie baking in the sun before cotillion. Mom wants me to know how to dance, so I go, but I always feel like a wallflower. She's hemmed up her voile dress, so that must prove she cares how I look. I know she must love me, but the other day when I told her I felt like the ugliest girl in the whole junior high and I wanted to die, she said, "Beauty comes from inside, Jo, *not* outside." In my head I screamed, *But Mom, please tell me I'm not ugly! After all, I am your own flesh and blood.* Then I reminded myself I was the only person in our family with green-blue eyes—everyone else has pure blue—as if it proved I don't belong. I ache to feel accepted. Instead I repeat what I often hear, "Buck up, Jo. Pull up your bootstraps and *quit* feeling sorry for yourself." I decide I *must* find some beauty inside. I excel at singing and sketching and remind myself, *if I do better, they'll care more.*

At fifteen I begin working in a greasy fried-chicken-place to earn money for contact lenses. With the removal of braces after being called "fang-tooth," and my newfound green eyes, a butterfly begins to emerge from its ugly cocoon. I smile shyly into the camera lens for my sophomore picture, pleased that my hair now grown to shoulder length, flipped up at the ends, will render this a photo I can finally give away. I nervously open the packet to find a likeness that actually makes me *smile*. I just know my family will be proud of it, and me, too.

But Mom announces, "It doesn't look like you."

"You look like a _____," Grandmother says, referring to another nationality.

The familiar prejudice and putting others down to build us up is suddenly very personal. I trudge to my bedroom. Tears of hopelessness cement my decision to toss them. I get my hair cut short after tiring of all the family criticism. I hate each photo until I work up enough courage to grow my hair out again no matter what is said.

Doubting I can ever be what my family wants, I pray to barely part the dark clouds with the letter I write to my parents:

"I've always given myself whole-heartedly to living and I've overdone because of this. How Christ died for me, the love he's given, the purpose for living I have, even with MS, is the highest reason for any involvement. My friend said she can't relate every MS attack to some form of stress, and we can stay home resting our whole lives and still progress with it. I'm excited to be learning—life isn't supposed to be stagnant and there's no room for bitterness. It's too great to be alive. Love, Jo."

I never hear a word about this letter or the book I send, which is *Joni*. Even though Ron hasn't read it, I've told him about her. I'm deep into Joni's second book, *A Step Further*[3] and it galvanizes my thinking. I want to live *looking* for what God wants to do in my life.

I don't complain during the attack anyway. My heart *literally* fills with song as I sit weakly on our piano bench. I've been reading Psalm 28 about blessing the Lord because he hears my prayers, and a tune flows for the verses. As I write out the melody in a round, it ends, "with my song I shall thank him," and I'm *actually doing* that very thing.

On a hot, sticky summer evening I feel too tired to attend Ron's Bible study. He comes home sullen, telling me he can't take *this* anymore. I ask, "What?" and he says, "You not being there with me."

I must not get weak, but I'm not supposed to overdo. How do I know when to rest and when to go? The mental gymnastics—cart wheeling in my brain—fatigue me further. I journal—"I want to give my life for others, but I can't or my health will go altogether! Use me as your servant, Lord. I yield my life to you."

Ron and I sit on the bench-seat of our Galaxy in the parking lot outside Dr. Black's office. My exam showed pronounced reflexes in both legs along with various other symptoms, but when I walked, Dr. Black said, "I think your gait is caused by emotions, not MS. Are you having trouble accepting the disease?"

While I look at Ron I say, "I think I have been building up a lot of anxiety." Ron says, "It seems natural because of the surgery."

"I've been afraid Dr. Black wouldn't want me to try it. MS patients have supposedly been helped—what if he didn't agree?" Tears fill my eyes. "Sometimes I'm afraid others, including Dr. Black, won't know how I really feel since lots of the symptoms are subjective and invisible—like fatigue. I'm scared they won't believe there's something wrong with me. I *hate* having this fear."

"Dr. Black just confirmed his diagnosis. He doesn't doubt it," Ron says compassionately.

I cry, "I don't want to make MS worse, Ronnie!"

As he turns the key in the ignition, Ron says, "I know you don't. It's okay."

I write in my prayer journal on top of Ron's prayer page (with my own shorthand for "thank you"—TU)—"TU God, for Ronnie—a wonderful husband, man of God, who loves me even with MS. Praise the *Lord*."

Six years later I will read "But You *Look* So Good,"[4] explaining how difficult it is for people with MS because of the silent, indiscernible symptom fatigue. We can look great though we might feel quite different. For me, the problem of being believed rises from a deeper level …

I'm a senior in high school. Mom's finally settling down in the upholstered rocker in our middle-class neighborhood filled with cookie-cutter-ranch-style homes. I tell her how painful it's become for me to sit on the wooden seats at school.

She says, "Don't be such a baby, Jo," and I berate myself for bothering her.

A few days later when I sit on the cushy, green and gold brocade sofa, Mom's hard-earned wall-to-wall carpet appears in my tear-clouded vision as I instantly rise off it, doubled over.

"I don't mean to complain, but I have this big bump on my bottom and I can't sit without it really hurting," I say, waiting to hear that I'm whining.

Mom heaves a sigh as her fingers search my tailbone.

I cry, "Ow!" and jerk away.

Shock registers on her face, "I'm calling the doctor tomorrow. There *is* a bump."

I don't know whether to cheer for being vindicated, or cry for fear of what the doctor might do.

As I lay on the examination table, Dr. Purcell lances the polyneidal cyst, then squeezes it while I fight back a scream and whimper instead. Mom stifles a cry herself, and I wonder *does she feel badly for not believing me before?*

Surgery to remove the cyst growing from my tailbone, no doubt bruised when I tobogganed that winter with boisterous friends, bouncing from snow-covered bump to bump, proves even more painful. A friend brings tiny bottles of vodka given to his parents on flights. It mixes well with hospital orange juice. *At least I didn't make it up.*

In California I undergo vertebral basilar artery insufficiency surgery, an experimental treatment for MS. It's supposed to allow more oxygen to the hindbrain where MS lesions are causing symptoms. I'm now able to sing solos without hanging onto something. Take short walks in our neighborhood with Jessie. And fix gourmet meals. Our church members are thrilled. Dr. Black is thrilled. So are we. Within a few months the improvement wears off, and MS attacks come and go like freak weather patterns, exacting their toll on my body like the damage of low-class hurricanes.

During church we sing, "When peace like a river attendeth my soul, when sorrows like sea billows roll, whatever my lot, thou has taught me to say, 'It is well, it is well with my soul,'"[5] while I cry silent tears. If Horatio G. Spafford could write such words from a ship at the very place at sea where all three of his daughters drowned earlier, how can I not claim it is well with *my* soul?

When I see Dr. Black, I explain I *was* anxious, and I don't want to make MS worse than it is. He's kind and understanding and I'm grateful. He suggests I continue the transfer factor, and possibly try another experimental treatment, immuran injections.

"Let's go to the Pizza Place!" says a young man after Bible study.

As we pile into cars I whisper to Ron how tired and off balance I feel, but he says he'll help.

"I'll help too," says our spunkiest teenage girl. I smile in the car's darkness.

I lean heavily upon these two arms and hear, "Ha, ha! Is she drunk or something?" A burly young man shouts loud enough for all in the restaurant to hear. Tears fill my eyes as we pass his booth precariously.

"I'm sorry, honey," Ron whispers.

I wish I could announce to everyone that I'm not drunk. *Help, Lord. I don't want to break down in sobs.*

I begin balancing with forearm crutches in the spring. After being dependent on others' arms for a few years, I welcome the aides. At least now I have a visible reason for walking so erratically.

Taking two classes at the seminary fills my mind with knowledge while my heart overflows with the joy of learning, diverting my thoughts too easily consumed with MS. It's a short interlude. After one semester I must quit, but I make a new friend, Marilyn, who comes often to our home.

After driving slowly to a women's meeting at church, I'm asked how I'm doing.

"I'm learning so much about how God uses suffering in our lives."

I do *not* say I recently journaled— "TU for the excitement I feel knowing every problem brings me closer to you, God." I'm not sure people would understand me feeling *excited.*

"Jo, someday you're going to write a book," says our senior pastor's wife.

"*Me?*" I answer doubtfully while looking into her smiling face. "I feel like I fall desperately short of how I should be living so often. It's an everyday-learning-experience, that's for sure."

"You're an example to me, Jo. I don't know how you do it."

"Well, thanks," I say as I sway off in the direction of my car, praying, "Help me learn all I can during life with MS, God. It's so much harder to praise you with this than Costochondritis."

Arriving home, I fold Jessie's long ears around my face, then lie down.

Ron opens the door, saying "Hi, hon," after making the hour-long drive from seminary in soft rain, which has turned into sleet. He kisses me and I ask about his classes.

I pray silently, *Lord, give me the words,* as I look at my fingernails nervously while Ron unloads books. It's so frightening to say things that are really important. When I'm this nervous my voice shakes and I sound even more anxious, sometimes agitated. What I'm really feeling is fear that what I'm saying isn't important enough to be heard, or accepted, or that I have a right to say it at all.

"I've been praying to trust the Lord with MS, and I know we pray together, but sometimes, like now, since it's been getting worse again, I'm afraid I won't be all you need in a wife. I just want to make you happy. It's what I've always wanted."

Tears threaten to run down my face.

"I know that." Ron reaches out his arms, and I sit on his lap.

After tender moments together I balance off furniture and walls to my sewing room to write in my journal— "Ronnie says not to worry about getting worse. 'We're in this together,' he said."

Anxiety melts away as if it is candle wax touched by the light of love's wick. *Together.* I remind myself, *together.*

Chapter 3

Weakened but Fighting, Learning, but Wondering

As we sit outside a McDonald's, I'm in a wheelchair we've borrowed for a day of sightseeing. We're carving time out of Ron's busy schedule for a date, since professors exhort students not to neglect their relationships. I feel grateful for how challenges with MS and ministry seem to be drawing us closer. I want that to continue.

In my peripheral vision I notice a young man writing on a small piece of paper. When he places the scribbled note in front of *me* as he passes by, I look up quickly with my eyebrows raised. It says— "If you go to so-and-so church tonight and confess all your sins, you will be healed."

"You're not going to believe this," I say as I hand Ron the note. "He doesn't know me, or how I want to live my life." It's not the first time I've been told sin could be causing MS. I've already been confessing every one I can think of.

When we get home I close our bedroom door, where I'm driven to my knees, pleading with God to reveal any unconfessed sin. I recall Jesus healing a man whose sin caused his paralysis (Matthew 9:2). I don't want to be like him. Suddenly, it's as if I'm under a waterfall cascading over me, cleansing me of dirt I'm unaware of. I feel *clean*. I remember another story of Jesus healing, this time a man who's assured that sin is not the reason for his blindness, but "that the work of God might be displayed in his life" (John 9:3). I know as surely as I know it's Tuesday, for the first time since my diagnosis, sin is *not* causing MS. I pray with moistened eyes, "I'm so glad I don't have to feel guilty for having this. I want you to get glory through it."

Then a seminary professor who believes God healed him of cancer exhorts me—it's God's desire to heal every disease. He tells me to visualize my body's good cells eating up MS-attacking cells, though no one knows what causes this autoimmune disease.

I see ravenous black-hatted cells trying to gobble up the myelin sheath. White-hatted ones rally together, mounting a defensive, counter attack, swallowing whole the angry black ones, and my central nervous system is relieved. I visualize this often, hopefully empowering my body to fight MS.

When Dr. Matthew's cancer returns, after he feels so sure God promised to heal, Ron and I feel shocked by a Richter-scale-earthquake. Then he dies, and we along with other students must acknowledge—whether we want to or not—that humans cannot decide how God's going to answer prayers. I realize Dr. Matthews *was* healed of cancer, for a time, and now he's totally healed—he's with God.

Betty, the director of the local MS Association, introduces herself to Ron and me, setting us instantly at ease. Her smile warms my heart and her gentle voice is enthusiastic. I had read an article in the newspaper about her perspective on dealing with MS, and I couldn't wait to see her. As I perform motions with my fingers, arms and legs, I can't help noticing MS has insidiously affected my nerves, which tell my muscles what to do. Betty believes through exercise I can help nerve pathways repair and resend proper messages to body parts. She gives me pictures of exercises I can do at home to keep from losing more mobility, and even build strength.

I'm eager to begin. I long to be stronger. I grieve not being able to hike in the mountains when we go back to see family. I used to carry a thirty pound pack into the high country. I'm honest about missing it, but encourage Ron to go ahead and have fun with the others while I sit in camp sketching, enjoying the smell of pine while watching blue jays and Clark's Nutcrackers flit about. I want Ron to continue doing things he loves. I allow myself to feel sad, cry, and write out my feelings. Through bouts of tears I ask God to show me what I *can* do. What I *can* enjoy. What Ronnie and I can do *together*.

And so I begin repetitions of exercises. Just when I attain a slightly elevated level of strength, inevitably a new onslaught of symptoms batters me back to ground zero. I sense God nudging me with courage, like a daddy encourages his baby to take each little step, and with each tumble, to get up and start all over again. Then I resume the snail-paced building of exercise repetitions—only to be hit once more. MS episodes attack me every few months.

As I recover I never know how I'll come out of the current attack. Will I be able to use my arms? Walk? Become bedridden? I know I can retain increasing disability with each "exacerbation," so I write at the top of my prayer requests— "I pray to trust God with my health."

Each time worry about what disability level I'll retain yanks me away from that prayer, it's as if a giant magnet pulls a tiny pin with ease. Through anxious tears I tell God, "I praise you," out loud. My heavy spirit invariably lightens as I take the focus off my fear and put it on the things I've been learning about God in the Bible. I can praise him because he is love—he proved it through Jesus' death for me. He is creator, and he created me. He is faithful, so he will faithfully use whatever happens to make me more like Jesus—if I let him—and that will bring joy into my life.

Then, I build exercise repetitions ... one repetition ... two repetitions ... five ... eight ... I can almost taste the sweetness of success. Muscle spasms jerk my legs up to my body in the evenings when I'm fatigued. I keep working to know what my body can stand. I even walk a short distance on our treadmill.

And, *again* exacerbated symptoms hit me. When the attack subsides, and the fatigue associated with it lets up a little, sometimes after taking dreaded steroids, I begin building all over again. One repetition ... three ... five ...

The meeting is to begin with a potluck, and the myriad of smells blend together into one potpourri. I stand behind my folding chair, wondering whether to hang onto chair backs to welcome others.

"Hi Jo, how are you?" says one of the cheerful ladies from our church.

I say, "Do you really want to know?" as I smile.

"Not really," she answers, turns and walks off.

Stunned, I sit and wonder what I've done wrong. Should I have said, "Fine?" At least I gave her fair warning that I'd like to tell the truth. I'm confused. Someone encouraged me just the other day to be truthful, "share the burden" with her because she cares. When I'm honest I feel guilty. I guess it depends on the person and timing. I need to not expect everyone to be interested. I need to learn how to avoid being hurt so easily ...

1976. Ron and I have been hoping I'll get pregnant, and though I stopped taking the pill years ago, it hasn't happened. We've prayed for days about whether or not to have tests my gynecologist recommended. I've heard when you *try* to get pregnant anxiety can actually block it.

My sister, Rhonda, and her family are in town, so everyone is at our house. The men sit around the living room laughing while women crowd in our kitchen preparing their own dish.

I remark, "We're trying to decide whether we want to go through all the tests to find out why I'm not getting pregnant."

"What's the hold-up?" says one.

"Either get pregnant or quit complaining!" another says.

I sigh inwardly. *I'm not complaining. I'm just being honest.* As I take white Corelle plates from the cupboard I decide to never bring this subject up again. Not with my family. They wouldn't know how to deal with my anguish each time a friend throws a baby shower. Both Rhonda and my sister-in-law, Marli, got pregnant easily. They wouldn't understand seeing the movie *Rosemary's Baby* terrified me. The young woman involved with evil people conceived a baby that looked like a demon! I announced afterwards loud enough for the crowd to hear, "*I'm* never going to have a baby." It came out like a vow I had to make, even though people stared. My family would laugh if I told them I wonder if I can't get pregnant because I said it—that I wonder *why* I said it.

It's 1980 and Ron now pastors a church. We live next door, with mighty oak trees spreading their canopy, where squirrels scamper from tree to tree, teasing Jessie as they race by. Her ears flap with every bounding stride, her deep bark resounding authoritatively. I delight in sitting on the porch watching God's brilliant red cardinals as they fly from perch to perch. Hummingbirds buzz near my head, as if in thanks, before they drink the sweet red syrup from the feeder. Contentment fills me in this serene setting I haven't felt since camping in the Rockies.

Kind and caring people have become my wheels since I can no longer drive. My legs are too weak to push the gas or brake pedals, and my arms can't turn the steering wheel. It's been difficult to ask for and accept others' assistance, but these friends show such compassion I'm realizing some people actually receive *more* than they give out. When I don't allow them to help, they tell me they're missing "a blessing."

We're farther from seminary where Ron now does Ph.D. studies, but he seems happy. I direct the youth choir by nodding my head. I'm also teaching a weekly women's Bible study. I sing solos as well as duets with Ron and others, and he and I give concerts where we share with audiences how we're dealing with MS. One of our favorite songs tells about praising God no matter what happens. Often, Ron reaches for my hand by the end of the song, or he puts it on my shoulder and squeezes. I sometimes quip, "If you must have a disease, you might as well have one that manifests itself uniquely in each individual," because MS does.

Dr. Black tells us he's seen a marked degree of deterioration in the past few months. My arm muscles quiver like leaves in the breeze. Sharp muscle pain draws my legs up in jerky spasms whether I'm tired or not, even though Dr. Black says there isn't much pain associated with MS. A spoon being stirred in a pan sounds like fingers scraping a chalkboard amplified one hundred times, so I clutch my ears. Patchy goose bumps cover my arms and legs. Vertigo keeps me from turning my head at all. These don't include neurological markers Dr. Black observes. He says the MS may have even evolved into the Secondary-Progressive type, which may not go into remission. He wants me to have treatments called plasmapheresis, where my blood will be removed and the plasma centrifuged off. Fresh donor plasma will be mixed with it and returned to my body.

Just before our drive to the hospital, I'm handed a book written by a woman famous for her healing ministry while told, "I don't know why people have expensive treatments when they could just ask the church elders to pray for healing."

I feel ambushed by criticism. Challenged again about what I believe. We've been praying for God to heal me, and others have prayed over me. I pore over my Bible while I await Dr. Black.

"Jo," he says, "I'd like to do another spinal tap so we can compare the results before the plasmapheresis, then after."

I ask, "Are you sure I won't have the same problem?"

He responds, "That's highly unlikely."

So I agree to it.

I lie flat for sixteen days this time, after two blood patches prove unsuccessful at filling up the hole that leaks spinal fluid into my back. During the long days I welcome visits from nurses and friends. Dr. Black doesn't charge me for his daily visits because he feels responsible, advising me *never* to have another spinal tap unless it's necessary to rule out spinal meningitis. Evidently the membrane that covers my spinal cord doesn't heal easily from a needle-prick-sized hole.

After it closes I lie on a gurney in an operating room under the scrutiny of the hematologist. He uncovers my entire body when he's ready to insert the large needle in my femur artery. I flush with embarrassment. *Why can't he see he doesn't need to totally disrobe me to insert a needle in my groin?* Why can't I open my mouth to tell him?

As I lie still for hours with needles in my outstretched arms and groin, terror suddenly grips me. I pray fervently to control the quickness of my breath and trembling. "Help, Lord!" I whisper. Immediately I see Jesus nailed to a cross. My heart wrenches—not for me—for him. His love seems to flow through my veins along with my blood being reintroduced. The panic attack's grip is loosened, and I drift off to merciful sleep.

The next day as I'm about to be released, a nurse who often cared for me, and often sneaked in just to talk, rushes in to say, "I just want you to know, Jo, even though you've had to be here so long because of the headache, I don't believe that's the whole reason. You helped me know God better! I *know* that's why you had to be here. I'll never forget you!" She squeezes me ferociously, as if her hug will make me believe what she says. It does.

While I recover from overall weakness due to lying down for sixteen days, I study the book about faith-healing. A flame ignites within me. Years before I'd noted in Bible margins all the healings Jesus performed, and the various reasons for illnesses and afflictions. Now I study those as well as his apostles'. Jesus evidently did not heal everyone, though he *did* heal every disease, and people were mentioned in parts of the New Testament who weren't healed. Then there was Paul, whose exemplary faith can't be doubted. He prayed three times for his "thorn in the flesh," whatever malady he suffered, to be removed. Instead, God told Paul that his grace was sufficient for Paul (2 Corinthians 12:7–10).

I discover God works in different ways in different lives. We can't *expect* out of God a standard operating procedure because he *is* God. Some are healed and others are not. If not, God *always* wants to use it to touch others' lives as well as the one who suffers. I hunger to understand what God wants to do with my life if I continue to have MS. I dwell on Romans 5:3–5:

> We also rejoice in our sufferings, because we know that suffering produces perseverance; perseverance, character; and character, hope. And hope does not disappoint us, because God has poured out his love into our hearts by the Holy Spirit, whom he has given us.

If I have to have MS, I want to live by the power of the Spirit with hope. I want to feast on any purpose God gives to the unpredictable life I lead. I do not want to merely survive MS.

After six plasmapheresis treatments Dr. Black can't detect any improvement. The hematologist puts me on the chemotherapy Cytoxan, but I develop massive hives. After going off and on it three times, the physician declares, "You must be allergic."

Looking back through journal notes I see how often I've prayed about which unproven treatments to try. I'm tired of chasing after them. I just want to be healed miraculously, or learn to accept *not* being healed. As if clouds of uncertainty part and a ray of light shines clearly through, I sense peace that God isn't going to heal me now, so I pray, "Then use it, Lord."

Bright spots in all the hospitalizations occur when people say they were touched by the strength God obviously gave Ron and me. Who say how inspired they were by Ron's devotion as he lay night after night on a cot nearby. Who tell me they came to know the love of God through me. I journal—"TU Lord for MS. Yes, Lord, I *do* thank you, because you're teaching me so much through this trial. I love hearing your Spirit speak to my spirit as I've slowed down. It's a treasure I never want to lose. And TU for how you're using MS in many lives."

Then Grandmother writes, and I know much of what she exhorts is true of me—I am spunky. I do sing and praise God when I feel down. I'm incredibly blessed—often writing out my thanks with, "TU for …" literally lists of things. But I blink back tears, doing the very thing she said not to do—cry. Though I love Grandmother, and we share a deep faith, I feel the same frustration with her I feel with the rest of my family. Why isn't it okay to be truthful at times, to admit an emotional, spiritual, even physical *struggle?* What makes being truthful wrong? I remember being told, "You don't have to tell *all* the truth, Jo," and white lies were common.

I pen a letter to God on March 5, 1981:

I really want to be willing to suffer if my testimony of how you give me strength in living with MS is better than a testimony of perfect health. Is that negative? It's scriptural according to Paul's experience, even though

I'd rather not have MS. At the same time I want to fight disease progression. To be positive so Ronnie doesn't get discouraged. To be a good wife and if you ever desire it, a good mother. How I love you and want to trust you and grow in humility and love and joy and peace. TU for being my Lord and Savior and Friend. Jo

Is it all the hospitalizations? All the experimental treatments adding up to zero help? The hives? I'm not sure what's causing Ron to withdraw, to look away with tightened jaw when I encourage another person with MS over the phone, but something is happening. I journal—"Ronnie would not be frustrated with the MS."

Chapter 4

Betrayed, Blamed, and Devastated

The months speed by. I unwrap my Christmas gift from Ron, reading aloud, "To my wife, IOU a day together doing whatever you choose! Love, Ronnie." Suddenly I realize I haven't asked for time because Ron's already overwhelmed. Because that's what wives of seminary students do—sacrifice—why else would they award us the "PHT (Put Hubby Through) Degree" when he graduated with his Masters of Divinity?

After taking a bus trip to Rhonda's, upon my return, Ron says he's never letting me go again. He doesn't like it when I'm gone.

One afternoon I shop and see a movie with Jean and Brian and their mother, good friends of ours. I feel like a child, laughing gaily as they twirl me about in the wheelchair, none of us the least bit ashamed.

When we get home around six Ron says, "Where have you been? I've been *worried*."

We take in a traveling exhibit of Masters' paintings at an art museum for my IOU. Ron kneels beside my wheelchair as we gaze admiringly at Renoir's *The Boating Party,* and I bloom like the painter's radiant flowers under Ron's attention. MS feels small when we're enjoying ourselves. We agree to do this more often.

"That was a good sermon," I say after Sunday service. Ron's so insecure, I want to build him as a preacher. He's asked me to pray for him. "Why don't you use that same approach more often? It was *really* effective."

Ron's face darkens. *What have I said this time?* His face masks his feelings, so I ask, "What's wrong?"

Ron states, "Nothing," but his cloudy mood continues.

He's fine after cloistering himself in his study in the church, so I don't ask anymore.

At breakfast I offer, "I'll be glad to go with you," because Ron feels uncomfortable making house calls. I open up immediately to strangers, like a door thrown wide to dear friends. Inevitably, I rescue him from the uneasiness I see creeping into his face by filling the silence when others expect him to speak. It didn't used to matter much, now Ron seems annoyed.

He states, "I *should* be able to do this myself."

"You have other strengths. Not every pastor visits homes," but he sighs.

In the late spring we take a carload of teenagers to a huge gathering in a nearby city. The auditorium resounds with the theme from the movie *Chariots of Fire.* My heart swells and I wipe at wisps of tears as runners enter the stadium track far below. The conference theme about running the race of life with Jesus pulsates with the steady beat of the song. Now I see runners pushing young men and women in wheelchairs, and tears escape my eyes as I pray silently, *I'm not alone. I'm helped along and I can 'run the race' with you whether I can actually run or not. I won't give up, God.* As Joni Eareckson speaks about her life with Christ, though paralyzed, I dab my nose and eyes with soaked tissues.

During the drive home an argument between Jean and Brian interrupts my ponderings. I see Ron looking in the rearview mirror. I hear his defense of Jean's position against her brother. I sense how unnatural and immature it is. I look back at Jean and see a plea that borders on something else. The look in their eyes fixed on each other sets off an alarm bell in my mind.

Later, as we watch Jessie's hopeless pursuit of gray squirrels I pray *how do I tell him, Lord?* I work to calm my voice filled with emotion.

"As I looked at you referring the argument, I noticed something. I know you care about being wise and careful. Jean seems to idolize you. She could easily misconstrue your attention."

Ron shakes his head in amazement, but thanks me for pointing it out, saying he'll be careful. *Thank you, God.*

Then Inga and Ruben, whom we met in Sweden, arrive. They thoroughly enjoy their visit, and later Inga writes:

"We felt so that Jesus lived inside you and that He gave you a special strength. Jo, I believe that God gives you a serene feeling He is planning something wonderful for you. Philippians 1:6: "He who began a good work in you will carry it on to completion …" Jo, I hope you can feel my embrace. We love you and Ron so much!"

In July, Ron and I head south for a vacation. After sight-seeing through several states, we attend a week of meetings to renew pastors and their wives. While talking with another couple, I hear Ron admit how much he wants children, but fears pregnancy would make the MS worse. I say I'll be glad to see my doctor. I feel bad for holding Ron back from his hopes for a family; that he hasn't been honest, as we'd promised. I haven't used birth control for years, though I've wondered if I could be a good mother.

After singing in the volunteer choir, I'm asked to sing a solo the last night. Sitting on the wooden stool I say, "Many of you have asked how we're able to have such peace and joy living with MS. Thank you for your concern. We have challenges, but I know some of you may have invisible problems. I've learned so much about trusting God because of having MS. His grace truly is sufficient when I tell him how I feel and how much I need him. He's been so good to me!"

I empathize with every line of a song of thanks, and tears fill many eyes as people rise to their feet in applause to God, because of who *he* is.

While Ron and I enjoy sumptuous Southern cooking, he says, "I'm falling in love with you all over again."

I know, as if his declaration was a letter to an editor—our trip has been good for us. Behind my spreading smile, though, is bewilderment. Has he felt *out of love?* Is that why he's falling in love *all over again?*

Back in the pastorate, life shifts into high gear, and our relationship, the slowest, away from eyes that spoke volumes when words of love were whispered in far away places of serenity. When we receive a letter from Klas my eyes tear-up:

> "I think of you quite often and remember the good times we had together … especially our prayer times together every night. Now, five years after my stay with you I fully realize how much it meant. You two really became good examples for me. Your love and kindness, your spiritual lives and your marriage have been a pattern to me."

The air conditioner runs full blast to combat oppressive heat. I hear the church office screen-door slam to see Brian striding down the sidewalk, as Ron approaches our house with his head so low it seems to rest on his chest. He sighs heavily as he drops next to me on the couch. *What in the world can be wrong?*

His voice rasps as he tells me Brian came to tell him in private he *knows* Ron is involved with his sister, Jean.

It feels like a knife stabs into my heart, while at the same moment I plummet down a bottomless, dark tunnel of despair. Spinning, spinning downward into a funnel that has no end, I fall, lost and out of control.

"Wha-t- I don't understand. I *love* you," I say, tears coursing down my cheeks, my shoulders now as hunched as his.

Ron says he *does* love me and wants to remain with me.

Then why—? Is it my fault?

He commits to work on our marriage, but says he's struggled with emotional love for me over the years and thinks MS has something to do with it, though I don't complain about it. He admits, at times, it disgusts him when I need to use crutches or the wheelchair. He's afraid God expects us to have such a testimony living with MS that I'll become paralyzed like Joni Eareckson.

I say, "We can't let fear take over, but instead encourage each other when one of us feels scared."

I ask Ron to see me as his wife who loves him, rather than a woman with MS.

He says he feels he's only known as the one married to Jo because when we're talking with others they're only looking at me. I was more gregarious than Ron when we married. Now it bothers him. When we sing together he only hears me being complimented and he's jealous. I ask if he'd like to quit singing duets. He doesn't answer. He tells me we've had good years together but our personalities are so different; it's hard on him. I've helped him change for the better, but he wants to be stronger and I'm a reminder of how far he has to go. I cry out to God:

> Encourage Ron, please. How can I create the right atmosphere for his love to grow when I feel so insecure and hurt? How do I act normal? What is normal? I've tried to please Ron and be what he wants, say things so they won't hurt him, and yet I still do. Oh, help me.

Three weeks ago Ron told me his love for me was growing, now he says he and Jean are still involved. It isn't because of lust; he wants to help her grow up because she needs him—she's insecure like he is. He goes on to say Brian knows about the love letters Ron sent to Jean. Ron wrote Jean that he loves her, and if he wasn't married to me … Brian's going to make Jean burn the ones she received from Ron. I'm slumped on the couch in agonizing physical pain—worse than any MS pain—the pain of betrayal. I even *warned* Ron. Somehow my mind kicks into gear while my heart is stuck in quicksand.

"Did Jean write you letters?" I ask in fear.

When he nods, I say, "We need to burn them."

Ron looks stricken. Jean, the teen who helps me shop. The girl I give voice lessons to because of love and the desire to build her confidence. Who helps me pack, even the trip where Ron said, "I'm falling in love with you all over again," not two full months ago.

I can tell Ron doesn't want to burn the letters, so I say, "If you mean what you say about wanting to work on our marriage, you know you can't keep them."

He nods in resignation, goes to his office and returns. I sit on the front porch in a stupor. I haven't even prayed. I just know in my heart we're doing the right thing as I strike a match and flames engulf the letters in a tin pie plate. The acrid smell of sulfur burns my nostrils and smoke clings to the muggy air like the memories Ron obviously holds dear to his heart, for they're painted across his anguished face. He does *not* want to cremate the vestiges of his liaison with Jean, and I feel a part of me incinerating.

"I don't know all of what happened, but I forgive you," I say. "I want our marriage to grow stronger than ever."

He tells me he really does love me—he tried to break it off with Jean three times—if I don't still want him, he'll die. Through tears bonding us together in pain, we commit to a weekly date to revive our study-and-ministry-starved-relationship, but after we go to bed I get up to write:

> God, is it my fault? How can Ronnie think I don't need him? I've grasped onto you and the Bible's truths so that fears, which well up within me regarding MS won't overwhelm me. If I hadn't, I would've shriveled up into a rotted grape, sour and bitter. The irony is, in my holding tight to you I appear so strong I don't need Ron, or so he says. Can cultivating a strong faith have its drawbacks? I can't let go of you, God.

We sit with a professor while Ron tells him about Jean. I blow my nose often.

The professor says, "It's only natural to be angry, Jo. Don't feel guilty, even though you forgive Ron. Ron, you need to *accept* her forgiveness. You have two choices—move away, or stay, but Ron, you must *promise* Jo you'll have no more one-on-one contact with Jean."

He asks if we want to come for counseling and though I do, Ron wants to come alone to work on his self-esteem. On our way home he says he'll keep that promise.

Since Ron drives to the seminary each Monday evening to teach, I ride along to attend hydrotherapy for people with MS. During my first session, I'm so excited to improve my condition, I overdo. I can't get out of the water. I hear Ron's disappointment—or anger— "Every time you exercise you have an MS attack. What's the use?"

"But I keep trying, that's what matters."

The following weeks I'm more careful, gradually building some strength.

One Saturday my shoulder hurts, so I apply analgesic cream. Within hours I break out in sores and I'm hospitalized, this time with a severe case of shingles. Cytoxan is blamed since it's known to cause the chicken pox virus, dormant in the body, to flare up. Ron doesn't stay in the hospital. He says the only reason he's done so was he didn't want to stay home alone, and he hates himself for it. The sharp pain of shingles forces itself outward while the knife wound in my heart throbs with every negative comment from Ron, thrusting inward. Tears wet my face, but I can't tell the nurses I know and love why.

Ron is nominated to the Outstanding Young Men of America.

We travel home so he can officiate for the funeral of a dear relative, and since we heard MS persons can ski, we decide to check out the National Sports Center for the Disabled at Winter Park.

I look up at the ski instructor and say, "I-I don't know if you can help me, but I'd like to try. I have MS and even with crutches my knees go out from under me and I fall. Can we make an appointment for tomorrow?"

"We'll have you up on skis in ninety minutes!" says Dave Clift, his grin surrounded by auburn mustache and beard, matching his full head of hair.

I'm *terrified!* Instructors, Anne Eckert and Dave, know what they're doing, though. The ski tips are connected by a piece of steel called a ski bra. And wedges of wood underneath the back of my boots force my shins into the stiff ski boots, changing my center of gravity so my legs won't collapse. Instead of poles they give me a pair of heavy outriggers, short skis attached to forearm-type crutches. A snowmobile waits to take me to the ski lift, but my feet bear weights. I sit and Anne lifts each heavy ski boot for me.

I'm so wound-up I sputter, "Tha-ank you."

Getting my gear put together at the ski lift is *nothing* compared to the thought of dismounting while it's moving. But Winter Park (WP) employees know to slow it to a stop if need be for disabled skiers. As Anne advises me, it comes naturally!

"Ohooooo, I'm skiing!" I yell. "Thank you, God!"

I lean into the outriggers to support myself, but after one traverse on the bunny slope I must lie down. At least the back of each outrigger has a serrated edge that breaks the speed to a stop with more leaning. Anne and I talk and laugh, getting to know one another a little more with each traverse and rest during the two days in which we ski an hour both mornings and afternoons. Ron and I had skied only a few times before MS. We share a special romantic evening and I'm excited as we consider a holiday ski vacation for next winter.

When we return, I see my gynecologist about getting pregnant. Since he adamantly discourages it, I call Betty. She gives me statistics proving pregnancy itself doesn't makes MS worse; it's when a woman doesn't have enough help with the baby. So, I change doctors and he discovers endometriosis might be preventing pregnancy. After that's surgically removed, I begin hormone treatment.

"In six months I can try fertility drugs and maybe get pregnant and we'll have a family, Ronnie."

He says if there were a contest of thirty-some-year-olds, I'd win. I feel like his queen.

But only for a day.

My glass slipper falls off as Ron learns more about himself. He confronts me angrily about domineering him. We never argued before. I didn't want to be like my parents so I always backed off, became quiet if I was talking too much, calmed down my enthusiasm if I was too excited, tried to figure out his needs and how I could please him. Ron's parents never argued, so I felt Ron's displeasure through his withdrawal, which left me feeling alone and *bad*. Now I face an *eruption*. Hot steam seems to vent from Ron as he realizes he was *happy* being weak, less than me as a person, and now it makes him sick. He feels manipulated by me in all ways, saying I overreact to everything.

My mouth hangs open. I'm totally baffled. I defend myself with, "I didn't know. I'm *sorry*."

Oh God, I must be a very ugly, unlovable person for Ronnie to have stopped loving me.

As months pass, I pray constantly for change within me to create change in our relationship. Then I discover Ron talking with Jean on our phone in soft, intimate tones. Though I remind him he promised not to do that and I'm hurt, he doesn't stop. The sorrow in my heart feels like the knife already inserted is now twisting, wrenching, torturing me.

One evening he says he doesn't know how he can trust himself with women as a teacher. While he returns to his study the bandage I continually apply to the wound in my heart blows off. I curl up into a ball with my arms encircling my legs and rock back and forth in our closet.

"If he can't trust himself, how can I ever trust him, God? Please take care of me."

I'm in junior high at summer church camp sitting around the campfire singing, then tell friends, "See ya' later," and wander away.

I hide in a bare patch among a circle of thick bushes. I want to die—I don't know why, as I sob, I just do. I rock to and fro, pleading with God, "*Please* let me die." Later, I sneak into my cabin feeling like a kitten in a litter of pups. I don't belong. The next day I put on my "happy face" with a smile as if nothing happened.

When my mother's best friend dies, I'm a senior. Her husband invites Mom to go through his wife's clothes to see if she wants anything. Since Mom grieves the loss of her girlfriend, I go along. I'm her friend's size, so I'm supposed to try things on. Mom wants me to wear them. To please my mother I go to school in her dead friend's clothing—styles no one my age would wear—feeling dead myself.

Ron's contact with Jean continues and I crash emotionally, harder than ever. Though the spring day is brilliant with sunshine, clouds of confusion and depression block the Lord's light. My world has grown dark and lonely. I don't know how to exist in it any longer. After more than two years of inability due to MS weakness, I've recently begun driving again. Betty thinks my off-kilter hormones, which have been affecting the MS drastically, are now evening out with the progesterone. Maybe God's just chosen to renew my strength. I lovingly nuzzle Jessie, telling her she's so special. Then I sit resolutely behind the wheel and back the car out of the carport.

I don't plan to return.

I don't think of it as suicide. And I don't believe killing myself will damn me to hell. I just want to go home to be with Jesus. He loves me. I can't stand the silence with Ron. The way he doesn't look at me, for his eyes seem devoid of feeling. I can no longer hope for change; Ron tells me I'm hopeless. He can't forgive me for *who* I am. He says it's just my personality.

"Lord, I'm swallowing some of the quicksand I've been sinking into. My very life is choking. Let me come *home*."

The straight country road allows me to accelerate. I near the curve forming the lip of a steep embankment ahead. I'll *propel* the car off the pavement. The impact will blow it up. My foot slams on the gas. *Faster and faster,* the car speeds.

Suddenly, it is as if God's hand takes the wheel and his voice says, *"No, Jo, I won't let you do this. I love you. I still have a plan for your life. Trust me."*

Sobs wrack my body as the car rounds the curve with a control that's not my own. *Trust. "Trust in the Lord with all your heart and lean not on your own understanding; in all your ways acknowledge him, and he will make your paths straight."* I memorized Proverbs 3:5–6 to help me with the uncertainty of MS, now they return to my mind. God's not calling me to himself through death. I drive home with a different resolve—empowered far beyond my own ability—to keep learning to trust God, no matter *what* that means.

Chapter 5

He Says It's Me, God,
How Do I Change?

Today I eagerly attend seminary chapel with Ron to hear a renowned theologian. After convocation, Ron wheels me across the charming campus to the bookstore where Carl F. H. Henry sits autographing books. Dr. Henry smiles and asks me if the wheelchair is a permanent part of my life.

"I use the chair for distances, and crutches, or balancing off furniture and walls otherwise. I have multiple sclerosis."

Dr. Henry tilts his head with compassion. "Use it as your pulpit."

I blink back tears, smiling. "I do. God's grace truly is sufficient."

Dr. Henry nods. Sneaking a peek at Ron as he turns the wheelchair, I sense his chagrin.

He tells me I act differently in public than I do at home so I have a credibility gap. Memories of our concerts—like balloons—rise above me and Ron's anger pricks every one. I really *believe* what I said, but with every new symptom I learn to adjust by being honest with God.

Ron says my credibility gap plays into the bitterness he knows he shouldn't feel, because he's just read Colossians 3:19—"Husbands, love your wives and do not be embittered against them." He says he needs to forgive me, but can't. No wonder I felt his hypocrisy Sunday as he preached about marriage.

I pray daily for God to change *me*. Perhaps *then* Ron will renew his love. One day I realize I want to change into the person *God* wants me to be. I pray to be more loving, forgiving, and patient as Colossians 3:13 exhorts. I claim that Christ is in me, the future hope of glory (Colossians 1:27). Ron wants me to make straightforward requests without underlying tones, manipulating, or lying about what I really want, then I read Colossians 3:9— "Do not lie to one another," and pray to communicate clearly.

When I ask Ron to study a book about marriage, we recommit to our own. I'm amazed to learn Christians can have a healthy fight—I'd always heard we weren't supposed to get angry. I don't want to argue, but I'm glad to know I should be able to express my feelings.

One evening after we've prayed for weeks about resigning the pastorate, then moving closer to the seminary after our upcoming trip overseas, I get angry with Ron. After praying I say, "I'm sorry for talking to you that way, Ronnie. I just feel hurt and jealous that if *I* express sadness, you feel guilty."

Ron says, "It was justified 'cause I'm being selfish and self-centered."

In the morning I awake, the room awash in sunshine, and Ron exclaims, "I *love* you."

Then for days he's withdrawn and I wonder *what have I done?* I keep trying to set my mind on God, not things happening here (Colossians 3:2), when I see Ron and Jean together. It's happening more rather than less. I pick up the phone and hear him speaking to her in hushed tones. My heart breaks all over again like a vase thrown to the floor. *How many minute pieces can it splinter into?* I tell Ron this doesn't help, and he says it's just *my* insecurity. It's tornado season, and I feel like a funnel whirls about inside me while Ron says he's confused about love. I turn to James, read, then write:

> Consider it pure joy, my brothers, whenever you face various trials of many
> kinds, because you know that the testing of your faith develops perseverance.
> Perseverance must finish its work so that you may be mature and
> complete, not lacking anything. If any of you lacks wisdom, he should ask
> of God … and it will be given him … Blessed is the man who perseveres

under trial, because when he has stood the test, he will receive the crown of life that God promised to those who love him, (James 1:2–5, 12).

God, thank you for this trial of living with Ronnie under tension because it's making me want to grow. This is the worst adversity I've experienced. I must trust when I ask for wisdom. I please you when I endure with joy, when I'm a supportive, loving wife, whether or not I receive any encouragement in return.

Ron pulls wide the door, and I walk awkwardly inside the mobility store. Against the wall stand two crutches, *unbelievably* light compared to my clunky, heavy ones with bulky, black forearm clasps and handles. These aluminum poles with thin gray arm and hand-rests in an ergonomic tilt *amaze* me.

I walk toward Ron saying, "Don't I walk more gracefully?"

"Well, I wouldn't say *graceful*," Ron answers, and my heart splinters a bit more, tears stinging my eyes. *Well, I feel more graceful.*

We fly to Sweden and stay with Inga and Ruben, seeing old friends. It's special to be here, but we hide our problems, and I ache inside with the secrets we hold, as if we carry signs—We are *not* who you think we are.

Upon leaving Stockholm we meet the rest of the archeological excavation team who've come to Israel from all over the US, having read about the dig in *Biblical Archeological Review.*

While sightseeing, I discover just how extraordinary these people are. Our tour guide tells me I can't go any further than the cable car stop on the side of Masada, but my new friends help me up those steps *anyway*. They literally carry me fireman-style across the huge plateau where zealot Jews held out against the Roman siege. Laughingly, they help Ron push and pull the wheelchair various places. Ron actually tells me twice during these days that he's *proud* of me.

Though I can only rise at 3:30 a.m. about twice a week to dig up pottery from the 10th century on the tell, I often work marking the "finds" of others, feeling useful and happy. I'm in the land where Jesus lived, died, and rose from the dead! But with Ron's jealousy, fear often whisks away happiness like a waitress retrieving an unfinished desert.

The young son of a leader forgets Ron's name so he says, "I might as well disappear."

"He's just a child," I answer.

At times I think we're actually growing closer, our love sweeter, at other times I wonder if it will all fall apart. Ron tells me he loves me occasionally and I'm so uptight with the confusion he feels about love I cry silently in bed. One day I write—"I want to be a quiet and gentle spirit (1 Peter 3:4) but with the friendly, bubbly personality you gave me. I wish Ron would be more confident so he won't feel I'm upstaging him or trying to be the center of attention, as he's accused me."

It's our last day in Israel, so I ask God to give me a way to express my feelings at the banquet. Suddenly words and a tune fill my head.

Later, I'm shocked to receive an award for my inspirational contribution to the team. I thank everyone shyly, then say, "I wrote a song of thanks for all you've done for *me*. It's called, 'And Then Come the Friends.'"

As I sing to Ron's guitar accompaniment, tears threatening my voice, I notice others are also tearful.

"And Then Come the Friends"

Some say life's not easy, some say life's not fair
Some people seem to have it all, and that without a care.
But what if life brings problems, pain and suffering
Some say it's time for giving up, but I say don't give in.
And then come the friends who make life easier
Who lift and carry ease the load, and make things possible
And then come the friends, who help me taste of life
Of places I've not been before, of more than I had dreamed
I wish to thank you friends for God's love shining through
A taste of life in Israel, made possible by you.
Life is meant for sharing and when we let them help
The increase of our joy is such that all can feel its touch.

So why not let them share it, let them come on in.
To share the thrill of simple things is God's design for us.
And then come the friends who make life easier ...
Taste of life by God's design made possible by you.[6]

Ron says later, "I knew you'd get the award," with the familiar ring of envy, and my throat tightens while tears pool in my eyes.

Crossing the border into Jordan, we travel south to Petra where I can ride a donkey! Red cliffs rise perpendicularly on either side, at times narrow enough to touch with both hands. The winding path leads through shadowy coolness when suddenly sunlight blares down, temporarily blinding our eyes before they fix upon an unbelievable sight—carved into the rose stone stands a *magnificent building*.

Shock registers immediately as stable hands gather each donkey's bridle. The lack of foresight and gravity of my situation aren't lost on my teammates, though. A couple guys step forward to offer their crossed arms, and I gaze upon monoliths carved 2000 years ago.

Unsettling fear closes over me at the flight gate, because there stands the young man who took care of Jessie while we were gone seven weeks.

When he says, "I had to tell you in person—Jessie was hit by a car and I found her lying beside the highway," Ron and I both begin to cry.

In bed, we sob, our precious dog's death opening floodgates neither of us knows exists.

We move to a rental near the seminary and within two weeks I've spoken for Ron by saying, "*We* think ..." instead of "I think," and he's furious. He says he's going to drive around before deciding if he wants to keep trying, or give up and get a divorce.

I kneel before Ron, tears dripping off my face.

"I'm so sorry I don't please or make you happy. I'll do *anything*."

Ron says he doesn't claim to be perfect, but in essence, he doesn't have hope or trust I can change and he's bitter that my identity's wrapped up in MS. My heart contracts as I replay his last words—"I know you don't like being called a hypochondriac, but what is MS anyway?" *How he could say such a thing?*

When he returns, Ron refuses to go for counseling, which I suggest. He says he doesn't want me fearing everything I do and say, but thinks we should live together and work on communication and being kind, and he'll just see if he wants it to work out. He doesn't think he can become all he wants married to me, and he selfishly wants that most.

From all I've read emotional love can die down and commitment brings a couple through the desert to an oasis of love again—but what if Ron isn't committed?

The next day I write—"Galatians 2:20 says the life I now live, I live by faith in you, Jesus. I need your nature and the fruit of your Spirit. I hate myself. Oh please, help me to change for you, me and Ron." Then I speak to Marilyn, who sees Ron at seminary, and she thinks Ron means *himself* when he says he doesn't think *I* can change. Yet I know I'm strong-willed, and sound like I'm right because of it.

Through a referral from Marilyn, I sit across from a counselor alone and say, "Please help me change my personality so my husband will love me."

Don asks, "What needs to change?"

And I say with hopelessness embedded in the answer, "Everything, I guess."

"I'm curious, Jo, what's the first recollection of you and your father together?"

What in the world does this have to do with Ron and me?

"I remember him taking me to an art store for a new sketchbook after my orthodontist appointment in junior high," I say, puzzled by my own answer. *Surely you can remember something before then.*

"What are the most important things you remember in early life?"

"My dad taking me to work with him on days it snowed so hard the school bus didn't come. Mom being pleased I spoke correctly at dinner and didn't have to be corrected like Dad often was. Mom's pride when I took the living-modeling course that taught me proper ways to behave. The shame I felt when my teacher ignored me, so I had to dart to the bathroom with diarrhea running down my legs in first grade. The anguish I felt every time my parents argued and I couldn't stop it."

Don says, "It seems you have difficulties with things you can't control. If you want your marriage to work, you'll need to keep from pushing Ron for a decision."

I pray all the way home—especially since a book on divorce lay in Ron's open briefcase this morning.

Sitting across from Betty at the MS Association, I blink back tears as I explain what's going on. She says fears are normal and I should be able to express them at home, but because of how Ron feels I need to be careful. She thinks the neurological textbook gave us too much information to ponder, and my parents' extremes about illness only caused more problems. She's excited about my taking a painting class, singing in the church choir, as well as continuing hydrotherapy. Betty gives me a booklet about Transactional Analysis, to help with my communication.

I read voraciously and realize, horrified, I speak like a parent to Ron! "You should" and "You need to," "You always" and "You never" are controlling and guilt producing statements. "Why don't you?" is accusatory, putting the other person on the defensive. "Wouldn't you like to?" is manipulative, rather than say, "I would like to, what about you?" I had *no idea* how I sounded. I heard this growing up. Oh, if *only* I'd known sooner. I suddenly see Ron's side, and it isn't until I'm changing sentence-by-sentence, thinking through what I say before saying it, slipping back into old patterns, apologizing, and rephrasing it, that I realize Ron does the *same thing.* But *I* want to change. It's so difficult to say, "I'd like to," "I need," "Would you please," because it means I feel valuable enough to ask. That my ideas are worth consideration. That I don't have to receive what I want.

Ron decides to see Betty at her request. As he tells how he feels, she suggests he appears to be in a mid-life crisis.

When Ron says he doesn't want that label, I respond, "But it kind of goes with what I've been reading—workaholic, avoidance and withdrawal from mate, and an affair. If you accept it we can have a really exciting relationship. Our communication is already changing."

He says he'll think about it, holds me on his lap that evening, then kisses and hugs me in bed before prayer.

He asks, "Was I good for you until this year, like you were for me?"

I answer, "Yes," tenderly; concerned this year will define our marriage.

During my next appointment with Betty I'm flabbergasted. When Ron told her the chief problem is bitterness about my credibility gap she asked if I ever claimed to be perfect. He had to admit, no. She told him our home is where I should be able to be me, but he put me on a pedestal—perfect—someone he could depend on. Now Ron's angry I'm not what *he* made me. When Ron told her how he feels about the attention I get because of MS, and he was angry I got the award in Israel, Betty asked if he'd rather I didn't go or try to do things on the trip or the tell. He admitted I should be myself. He felt it was wrong I got attention when I taught Bible study and led the youth choir and she asked if he'd rather I didn't do those either.

Then Betty asked, "Do you realize the position you've put Jo in? She can't please you if she *doesn't* do anything *or* if she does."

When he said he's jealous of people knowing me at seminary, she asked, "Did you try to form relationships there?" and he admitted he hadn't.

Ron said I always have something wrong with me.

As he described each one, Betty answered, "Those are real physical problems, Ron. Jo didn't make them up."

"Jo," Betty says as I sit slumped in despair, "He put you on a pedestal and that's why he compares his spirituality to yours and feels judged by you, even if you're not judging him. He says he came to seminary because of your exuberance and that's his responsibility, not yours. Ron can't fix the MS, so he wants to deny it."

I drive home thinking, *These past few months he said he loves me and cares about me, though he doesn't mean it the same way I do. Nowadays he reminds me we began our relationship for the wrong reason, anyway.*

Our first date is Halloween. He's quiet and gentle, yet fun, like Dad, and we desire to backpack in the mountains. We share a sensitive love for music. He "hides" in his pop/rock band behind the drums.

Soon after, a folk-band leader asks me to audition for their group losing its female singer. Our band had been their warm-up act at a club. I really like their sound and they perform the ski resort circuit so I'm excited. But Mom discourages me, saying Ron might not wait. *I wouldn't want to lose my chance,* deciding not to audition.

Ron and I announce our engagement in the club where his band plays. I so desperately want to be loved like the song "Cherish" sung by The Association. I think I've found that in Ron. Our relationship is hot and heavy, but I have to be a good girl like Mom says—I always stop anything before we go too far—I have to.

Now Ron has stopped making love. He says it doesn't mean the same thing to him that it does me. I come home one day to see him hanging up the phone. *Oh Lord, I suspect he's talking to another woman, maybe Jean. I thought they ended it months ago and he can't seem to forgive himself.* Four days later Marilyn tells me she thinks Ron's projecting into another relationship what we've been reading in the book about romance. She thinks, either in his mind or physically, he's carrying on a relationship with Jean, hence his guilt about sex. I cry, "Lord, would I be able to forgive again? I don't want to believe he's involved with someone else. I can only love unconditionally with your Spirit in me."

One night I get up from bed and journal:

> I feel like punching a wall! I could hate Ron for what he's doing. I'm mad
> and scared. I can't lie in the same bed. I feel vulnerable if he sees me naked
> because he's rejected my body and soul. "Help Jo as she waits for me to
> make decisions," he prayed before going to sleep—and I feel miserable
> and ugly and unloved. I want to yell, "It's unfair!" but that would push
> him away. Please give me hope. I pour out my heart to you for you are my
> refuge (Psalm 62:8). If I couldn't I would curl up and die.

After consulting with both Betty and Marilyn, I decide to speak with Ron about MS. "I asked Betty whether our fears could cause MS to worsen. She said when people are in a cycle of frequent attacks their anxiety level—

fear of future attacks—remains constant, and it *might* bring enough stress to exacerbate MS, but it wouldn't have caused all the attacks, and there's no way of knowing if it did at all. The way we were expected to be a testimony kept us from feeling we could be afraid and help each other deal with it."

Ron says, "Do you *deny* feeling like a martyr?"

"I did at one time, then realized I really did want God to use it. It's okay to feel fear, and I've talked honestly with God about it and grown *because* of that. *Jesus* was fearful in the garden of Gethsemane. I am *not* going to feel guilty anymore for being human about MS." I pause and look into his stoic face. "I'd like you to decide whether you want me to be The United Way poster girl since Betty asked."

Ron says if I want to, go ahead, but I answer, "You want to be assertive so I want you to decide because you're the one who feels I'm focusing too much on MS."

He tells me if I want to do it and have my name in caption, go ahead.

I respond, "There won't be any personal information on it, only MS."

The poster comprises a huge photo of me smiling in the pool as water drops from my arms raised in joy. Behind me, on the pool-side sits a wheel-chair. The caption says, "Making the least of MS—and the most of life." I unroll it for Ron.

"The only reason I did this is to help people, but this is how I want to live, Ronnie—reaching out to taste everything. That's why I wanted to go to Israel. No matter what you think, I never gave up."

I think Ron has teary eyes when he says, "I know. I'm not upset."

I'm wearing my t-shirt we bought at a fair recently. I wonder what the MS Association logo means to him—You Only Fail When You Fail to Try.

I feel *bitter* this morning. Ron said he feels cheated because he doesn't love me like he wants to love someone. I yell, "You say you won't allow me to be tested more than I can bear, Lord, *help*. Is it your will for my heart to be torn to shreds? I thought you were *for* marriage. Why, Lord? Why are you letting this happen?" my fist raised high in the air. Tears pour as I continue, "I'm asking but I don't expect an answer. I'm just glad you're not angry with me for having these feelings."

One of the profs I counsel with says, "Don't feel guilty if your marriage fails. You've been changing and you've been committed. Hope not only in your marriage, but even more, base your hope in God and his beautiful plan for your life even if Ron fails God *and* you." That afternoon, with fresh tears pouring, I journal—"I believe you love me and will take care of me, Lord."

Betty says a couple commented about how great I look on the poster. I feel so ugly to Ron, I soak up any compliment like a dried out sponge. One evening he fills the room with more negative statements. It seems they bounce from one wall to another, echoing, taunting me.

I say, "Don and I have been working on my self-esteem which is this small," my finger and thumb pinched almost closed together, "but it's growing."

Surprisingly, Ron nods.

"If you leave me, I'll make it. I'm a survivor, whom God loves, and he still has a plan for my life, but I *want* us to work this out. Our love can grow from ashes, extinguished cinders. When you told me the night you gave me our living-together-while-you-decided-about-our-marriage-terms, I said, 'I'll do anything.' I won't say that now because I realize I'm valuable to Christ. I battle to believe it, your rejection is so intense, but the Bible says it's true. I tried to become a nothing to build you up and you didn't like that either. I believe we can still grow together and have a wonderful marriage with God's help."

Ron tells me he doesn't believe in absolutes—especially about marriage.

Then he says, *again,* "I don't want to attack you as a person, so I can't say what it is except just things *in you.*"

I sit still, nearly paralyzed with grief.

Two days later Ron's angry again—he wants to live alone, that's the only way he'll know himself. He doesn't think we can be happy together and be ourselves, and he can't become all he wants married to me.

I ask, "Are you saying you want to leave?"

"Yes."

"Then *leave*," as I throw his jeans at him while he stalks away. I yell, "Yes, I *wanted* to hit you because you're hurting me so much since I love you so."

I shake like a leaf on a tree battered by a windstorm.

He throws clothes in a bag and heads out the door. I stumble around the house frantically. *What am I going to do?* I call the professor who counseled Ron and he says in answer to one of my statements, "If Ron says you domineered him, he let you. It's not your fault, Jo. We just have to pray he thinks things through."

I call Betty, who says, "Jo, one of the things Ron said about his romantic love dying ever since you've had MS, at the same time he has an affair, has concerned me. He's acting like other husbands who leave MS spouses. It's not your fault. I'm here for you."

Then I call a seminary student's wife I've become close to and she drives over to hold me while I weep uncontrollably.

Ron lives in a motel, but calls to share his tumultuous concerns about how the dean will talk when he must resign his Ph.D. in person. He wants compassion and I give it. He takes me to church and holds me when he brings me home, saying, "I'm sorry, I'm so sorry," while he sobs. He calls again to say he's interviewing with the company he left six years ago.

I say, "I love you and I'm praying."

Ron says, "I love you and care for you."

I don't know what that means to him. I sit staring at the walls after we disconnect. My life is incomprehensible.

In a few days he calls telling me he's found a place to live, "on the second floor."

I ask, "Is that for you or us?"

He says for him right now. My pain is so great I can't respond. He tells me to not worry about money, he'll make sure I'm okay.

"I don't want to live with my parents. I need to live by myself."

He understands. I sob till my eyes swell shut.

After friends help us pack, Ron holds me, pecking my cheek.

I cry, "I'm dealing with a lot of anger about this and my future, but I love you so I'm going to try to give you some time."

"I know that. I'm sorry this hurts so much because I care."

Mom flies out to help me drive back. On the way she listens compassionately for awhile, then begins to speak her mind.

My hands gripping the steering wheel, I say, "You said to me not long ago, 'It takes two, Jo.' That really hurt because I'm taking responsibility for my problems, and I *still* want our marriage. It only takes one to end it, Mom, and Ron can do that even if I don't want it."

Later on I say, "While I lived away I've felt blamed by you and other family members for having MS attacks. If I sense that, I won't let any of you know when they occur. I don't need that guilt." It's taken so much courage to speak up to her.

She answers with a manipulative, "*Okay, Jo.*"

When Ron and I painfully divide up things it seems as if it's forever. I feel like fourteen-plus years have been wasted. *No, I can't believe that.*

Chapter 6

Alone and Broken but Telling Myself the Truth

Inga writes in her letter exactly what I feel:

> "When one hour has went since we talked I said to Ruben, 'I think I have had a terrible dream. It can't be true. Did I talk with Jo?' We didn't know why it could happen. I am now thinking of David in Psalms 40:1–2. He was sometimes so depressed but the Lord raised him up. It will be for you, too, Jo. It's so hard to find words—even in Swedish. We can see that Ron has had almost the same hardships as you. We pray Ron is coming back and can love you for what you are in yourself again. We love you as our daughter, Inga and Ruben."

Inga's "Swinglish" brings a smile to my face even though I'm crying.

Thanksgiving nears without my feeling thankful—waves of sadness crash over me, one upon the other as I replay Ron's words. He doesn't want to spend the holiday together.

I wear long johns beneath sweats to keep warm in the bright, cozy one-bedroom apartment I'm renting as I read *Telling Yourself the Truth*.[7] I hunger to glean every kernel of wisdom. Three feet of snow cascade quickly from the shale-gray sky, mesmerizing me with the stark beauty of the blizzard. I can't help thanking God for this *gift*. And he blesses me during this and every subsequent snowfall by my thoughtful neighbor clearing a path in the sidewalk to my car he has cleaned off and dug out.

A book about marriage explains that a wife must *not* be a doormat, or she doesn't allow her husband to become more like Christ. I journal:

> As an assertive person I don't need to manipulate or dominate or blame. I need to be genuine, not a martyr or a stoic. My self-esteem is developed by accepting your unconditional love, God; developing a realistic self awareness (Romans 12:3) by completely accepting myself. Then I can see what needs to change, accept your forgiveness, and let you work in me. I now know we don't make another happy, each chooses to be happy. But I miss Ron so badly. I'm afraid, though your love removes fear (1 John 4:18). How do I grasp that? It feels as if life is nothing alone. Please fill me with your presence. Help me live for you no matter what.

A 1960s tune about a person wondering how nature can continue doing its thing when life has *ended* because his loved one left has played in my head for days. I need to stop the turntable.

With snow glistening in the sunlight on another day, I sit in my rocker and write:

> Psalm 62 tells me to rest in God. I must listen to you in silence during these lonely times, not just call someone, waiting with stability and confidence (verse 2). As Isaiah 40:31 says, I need to be a line twisted with you, God, to exchange my weakness for your strength. If I wait on you, you'll give me freedom of flight from fears and pressures. I'm helpless without you.

One day when Ron calls about picking up a blanket I say, "Though I've taken responsibility, I haven't asked forgiveness."

After I sincerely bring up each area, Ron says he knows I go over and over things and it's terrible for me, and he's sorry. He says I may not have learned this any other way.

I say, "Everyone makes mistakes. Please forgive me," but he doesn't, and I feel like I'm in the boat pushed out to sea again.

When I invite Ron for dinner to wrap gifts we bought in Israel he surprises me by saying, "You look pretty."

He *complimented* me?

"Thank you for what you said. I don't want you to think I don't forgive you just because I can't express myself."

We kiss and laugh before the crackling fire, teasing each other, reliving old memories, with more kisses as we say goodnight.

One day at a time, I tell myself, journaling pages. I discover I'm smiling at people, being kind to a clerk who makes a mistake, wishing I'd encouraged someone with a friendly attitude. The next day I'm thankful for the Bible study I attend, but I don't feel as joyful—I felt flattered by the guy in the car stopped next to mine who smiled and nodded. I realize I *crave* attention, though I don't think I deserve it. Then I read *no one* causes us to sin. An individual acts on his own. Ron told me once I *caused* him to get involved with Jean because I pointed out her interest in him. *He just passed the buck. I was an honest wife warning her husband of danger. I* must flee temptation. The final pain will erase any pleasure.

I feel resentment burgeoning within me like a boxer preparing for a fight. How *dare* Ron say I might not have grown any other way? If he'd told me years ago I would've gotten help and changed. I know deep down our marriage wasn't a sham. I wasn't *in charge.*

> God, is it fair I have to live in fear of what he might do? You have a plan for my life and can make my favorite verse happen for *me* no matter what Ron does—"And we know that in all things God works for the good of those who love him, who have been called according to his purpose" (Romans 8:28). What about *now?* Why should a man get to reevaluate his marriage to decide if it's what *he* wants?

My anger spent, I put away my gloves and remember to tell myself the truth—"You were rejected, you know how I feel." Then I cry, "But Jesus, you were never *married.*" Swallowing sobs I recognize more truth, "You were rejected by your *Father God* when you hung on the cross for *my* sins—a rejection much deeper than I could *ever* feel. And besides, to be rejected isn't the worst thing. *You* will never reject me." My list of truths continues:

> God loves me; he will hold me now, just as he has throughout MS; my personhood is in Christ, not in being Ron's wife; my success is in God—living life as Jesus would if he were here. Waiting on God. Drawing my strength from him when I have none. Letting him make something beautiful through rejection. Persevering with loving patience and overcoming this hurdle joyfully. Experiencing this trial without despair. Suffering this loss without bitterness.

But my emotions are hard to control. When Ron tells me he won't spend Christmas with me, tears escape my eyes.

I say, "I'll miss you," and he says the same. Sniffing, I continue, "I don't understand. I get very depressed at times, but don't love you any less."

I wipe tears covering my cheeks. He says he doesn't expect me to understand why he needs this time alone. He reaches for me and holds me tightly as he kisses me.

On New Year's Eve I sit alone and pen:

> I will stand, Lord. I'm one of your faithful. As in Job's life, you're allowing this trial sent from Satan so I can learn and grow in trust. Your truth will finally prevail. My loneliness, loss, sorrow—these are disciplines—your gifts to drive me to a life overflowing with you I might never have experienced otherwise, and *others* can be touched. Help me not become bitter and give the devil an opportunity (Ephesians 4:26–27). God, bless 1984, and I thank you painfully, with the sacrifice of praise, for 1983.

On Wednesday evening I attend the church choir rehearsal cautiously. Songs of hope fill my eyes with tears, and my heart aches with unfulfilled longing.

During prayer time I say timidly, "I'd appreciate prayer that my husband will return to our marriage." My tears flow unchecked as comforters surround me, assuring me of prayers.

Again, I sit in my special spot seeing more glittering snow, smiling in thanks to God. I pray to learn from the book I hold, *Love Must Be Tough*[8] by Dr. James Dobson, but my heart sinks as I absorb it.

> Ron's felt trapped, probably ever since I've had MS. He lost respect for me. He also felt entrapped by seminary and the pastorate. I've done something right—not calling or writing, but I've done wrong—by telling Ron I feel depressed and don't want to go on living I lay a guilt trip on him. I feel humiliated that I begged him to stay, saying I would do *anything* to keep our marriage—the very thing many spouses do when the other threatens to leave. I'm sickened to realize I was too lenient. Ron probably lost *more* respect when it was easy to continue contact with Jean. Dobson says that the trapped person feels better when their spouse sets boundaries about what they can tolerate—that shows confidence and self-respect that was lacking. Oddly, that may draw the straying spouse back. I need to show self-confidence that I believe I can make it with God no matter what Ron decides. Dobson suggests unless the relationship is already hopeless, this can bring a man like Ron back. But there may also need to be a time to bring up accountability.

Marsha and Jeff, who moved back a couple years ago, support, encourage, and counsel me. Other old friends shower me with love. They also reach out to Ron. Though he accepts invitations, he's unwilling to discuss us.

Even as I wonder if it's wise, I invite Ron to dinner when he brings the monthly check. He asks how I am and I say, "Doing well," matter-of-factly, proud of how I sound.

He asks about my physical therapy, which I can't continue due to the cost, then says, "Insurance companies should *encourage* that."

I'm *amazed* he's speaking with me about MS. Ron brings up his lifelong problem with assertiveness affecting him at work, then he reaches his arm around me, says he's really proud of my painting, and kisses me. We're cheerful in our goodbyes. *What's happening—is he growing?*

It's mid-January, and my fingers fidget while I wait for Diane to invite me into her office at the counseling clinic. I'm nervous about the personality test I took.

I go home with Diane's admonition, "*Quit* trying to change yourself. Ask God to search your heart, and to see if there is any hurtful way in you (Psalm 139:23–24). If he doesn't speak to your spirit of wrong, then *don't* worry and fret."

I actually *know* some of my strengths and weaknesses. I haven't *snowed* people like Ron's inferred.

Yet my confidence ebbs and flows. I call up Anne Eckert, who gave me her phone number at Winter Park (WP) last year. Her aqua eyes smile with her whole face surrounded by soft blond hair, and we laugh freely over Baskin Robbins ice cream. She says she's so glad to be my friend. I tell her I wonder why so many people care.

"Jo, you're the sweetest person, and fun to be with, and you have such interesting things to say. I can *learn* from you."

I thank her, saying she's fun too, and I look forward to skiing with her.

Today, as I visit Grandmother, I kiss her wrinkled cheek. She's ill and I love her so much. When she learned about Ron, she wrote that she *knew* how bad I felt. She tells me she never wanted to remarry after her husband left her with two little girls. She never felt she could trust any man again. I feel sad and concerned I could become distrustful.

One day I hear a radio preacher say, "If your husband is having an affair, ask yourself what you did to push him into the arms of another," and I sob with my face in my hands. Then I blow my nose and remind myself all over again the truths I've been learning, point-by-point.

On Valentine's Day I feel unloved by Ron, but God loves me. God's love is the *only* thing I can trust and believe in. Ron only comes once a month with a check now. If he calls I think I'm speaking clearly, yet he still claims I'm manipulative. I journal a list of TUs—Marshall and Judie's call and all the friends who care, adding:

> TU for the rides and great skiing with Anne, Dave and others; that I'm excelling, and it doesn't hurt as badly and I don't feel as stiff afterwards. I say, "It hurts so good," because I love it so. TU that it's so inexpensive for the disabled at WP, or I couldn't go. I'm learning from my mistakes,

the future is new, ahead of me. You're a God of blessing, and I will see it in the land of the living (Psalm 27:13). But God, I miss Ronnie so. Does he *ever* miss me?

After Anne and I ski one bright Saturday, I journal an entire page of things for which I am grateful, ending with:

TU for life—I'm *glad* I'm alive. For the condition the MS is in, and *isn't* in. Lord, I think it might be dawning on me. I've been claiming James 1:2–4, I Peter 1:3–9, and I Peter 2:20–21 to consider it joy to be going through this terrible trial. I think your Spirit is speaking to me—"*It's true Jo, you are growing through pain. This is not a limbo state.*" I resolve not to resist anything you wish to do in my life, though painful. I can be patient now because my life is *not* on hold. I'm living it *now*, through your power. I hurt. I fear. I get angry. I grieve over what is gone, and what *can* be lost. But I rejoice in you—who you are—God the Father, Son, and Holy Spirit; and in who *I* am—your beloved *child*. I seek above all else to reflect your glory so others see the power is from you (2 Corinthians 3:18, 4:7). I'm "sorrowful yet always rejoicing" (2 Corinthians 6:10). Father, I'm so glad to be *your child*.

I'll do *anything* to ski. I ride in a van-full of youth from church, ski with Anne, have so much fun I yell at the top of every run, "*Let's Boogie!*" and see so much improvement I yell, "*Thank you, God!*" I feel like Eric Liddell, the Scottish Olympian, felt about running, when I ski—God is *pleased.* It's a spiritual experience—a freeing of myself so I feel one with God's Spirit—soaring as an eagle. One day is all I should really ski. If I try skiing a second, I'm wiped out, much less coordinated, and hurting. But when I ski that first day, I don't feel clumsy, I feel *graceful.* Whomever I ski with has to listen to me talk about God's love for each of us. It comes as naturally as breathing in the pristine air surrounding me, and just as I must breathe, I must tell. And people listen.

While descending Berthoud Pass we hear on the radio why we're creeping along—a *250-car-pile-up* on the highway. Our driver detours into a tiny mining town and we pile out at a local historic church. I pick the spot under the altar as if I'm laying my life *on the altar.* I find myself praising God that I'm able to pray for Ron without frustration, fear, or bitterness. I thank God for the joy of knowing his peace, presence, acceptance, and love.

During prayer time tonight after choir, several thank God for the testimony I am *to them* as I handle this trauma, and I'm astonished. A friend says he sees a sparkle in my eyes and knows I'm doing better. I know it's Christ in me, for my emotions run all over the place and must be reined in almost daily to lovingly pray for Ron.

Angela, who leads MS hydrotherapy, believes I should use both crutches to conserve energy lost due to lack of coordination, and to steady myself for protection. She recommends me for classes offered by the National MS Society to train peer-counselors. I sit through each remembering how Betty tried to help me see I'm like others in how my self-image and self-esteem were hit. I'm also like others who feel guilty to be *relieved* to have a diagnosis.

Every day becomes more precious. I urge each friend—keep praying for Ron to return. Marilyn cautions me though. She's afraid Ron hasn't told me things that could surface later and hurt me *and* us. I journal—"Lord, Ron told me he and Jean were never sexual, was he lying? Should I ask Marilyn more? I don't want to."

"Oh God, Mom dropped it in my lap—Ron did *not* have his wedding band on when he brought the income tax return for me. I feel fearful *and* angry."

My family's rage at Ron flares while I recommit to our marriage. Ron's parents remain supportive and loving. When we last spoke I told his sweet mother, whom I've always called Momma, "I won't give up. I still love him." She said, "I don't know how."

In answer to my hurt about Ron not wearing his ring and my proclamation of love she says, "It would be better if you didn't. It wouldn't hurt so much."

I feel a new ache—are they losing hope?

On May 8, Ron calls, asking to come over so we can talk. I wonder if he's ready to do something serious—divorce? I remind myself God won't desert me. When Ron arrives I tell him excitedly what I learned in the MS peer-counselor training, and that I've been accepted as a peer-counselor. Ron seems to show a flicker of respect on his face as he says he's glad.

Then he explains he knows the world needs Joni Earecksons, but he can't be one. He couldn't take the pressure of other peoples' problems in the pastorate—he snapped. He says my zest for living is a problem for him—always would be—like when we were in Sweden and Israel and I got attention because of it. He'll always feel like I'm the more vivacious one people attach to—our friends are really *my* friends, not his.

I say, "You once appreciated and loved these qualities in me. Maybe you feel like this because of the way you feel about yourself. No one can get through to you how wonderful you are but God."

He says we're so different. I'm black and white, decide fast; and he's gray and thinks slowly and feels guilty he's not like me.

I grin and say, "I just read that very scenario in a book. It said we don't have to change or feel guilty or judge. We can rejoice in our differences, and see how they complement."

Ron tells me he's been angry for months about the money situation and I say, "I've offered to have you give me less, but you said it's your decision. I tried to give you respect and honor by letting you lead."

I begin to cry, "I'm not trying to manipulate you with tears. I'm just frustrated."

Ron says he never looked at it that way.

"I asked my counselor about something you claimed was manipulation. As long as you look at things through your filter, you'll expect and take everything that way. She says I can't win with you."

Ron nods. He's built up more irrational bitterness over the past seven months. Now he repeats I have a credibility gap.

Ron asks if I ever saw a lawyer.

"No, have you?"

He nods.

"What for?"

"Divorce."

My mouth and shoulders sag, "Are you still opposed to going to a marriage counselor of your choice with me?"

Ron looks down, "I don't know."

"Ronnie, I did not force you to love or marry me, and I cannot coerce you to return. It's your decision. I know what I want. I have a lot to offer and think I'm a pretty good catch." *Thank you, God.*

Ron looks at his hands as he says he doesn't know if we can restructure our whole lives and communication.

I answer, "We already have to some degree. I believe in me and you and *us.*"

He sighs, "It takes two to believe."

I'm teary as he goes to his car and returns with divorce papers I refuse to touch.

He says, "Hon, if we decide to work on this, we'll have to agree not to worry about everything we say. I'll think about going to a counselor with you." He smiles as he reaches to hold me.

I say, "Okay," as I hug him.

As soon as the door closes I journal:

Lord, he called me hon and I called him Ronnie. But I want to be encouraged to excel and reach for the stars—you've given me these desires. I've tried in the past few months to claim my marriage like I heard—if it's your will and I ask for it I can have it—John 5:14–15. What about Ron's free choice? I don't understand. If I could believe you'll make Ron come back, I'll wait forever. I doubt Ron, not you. My respect for him is dying. I pity him and feel angry that he let himself get like this.

A weight sits on my heart, then I recommit to my marriage and God lifts it off me as I feel his arms wrap around me in a soothing hug.

A week later I actually pray, "TU for this separation. You've used it to teach me who I am in *you,* who I am with MS, and who I want to be—free to be me." A few days later I pray, "I think, oh Lord, I've finally reached the point where I *believe* you have a plan for my life, with or *without* Ron. I can and will go on." The next day I pray, "TU Lord, you're still in control and I can trust you. You have a good plan for my future" (Jeremiah 29:11–14).

While I sit reading a few evenings later, Jean's mom calls. I barely understand her, she's so distressed—Jean is telling others about her affair with Ron. I *must* contact Marilyn and ask what I don't know. Eventually I'm put in touch with a pastor Jean talked to. Each of my friends agonized over whether to tell me what they knew. I now understand God's perfect timing—I would have been utterly crushed like a stomped pop can if I'd known sooner.

As Pastor Michael begins to detail Ron and Jean's affair, bile rises in my throat. I fight the urge to vomit as he reveals sordid secrets. My body shakes and I sob in disbelief, then disgust and hurt. Ron told Marilyn last fall before our move that Jean would wait for him—she loved him. Their plan was for Ron to divorce me and marry her. The confession Jean told Michael upset him so much he went to the dean about Ron, so when Ron resigned his Ph.D., the dean told Ron to leave the woman and go back to his wife.

Ron said, "I can't promise you that," turned, and walked out.

Michael, his voice exuding compassion, says, "It's no wonder Ron's been so ugly and blamed you for everything. He's felt guilty as he continued the affair. It's over now. Jean's dating someone her own age, even though Ron called recently."

I hang up the phone and weep, holding my stomach as I fold over at the waist, rocking, praying, "Father, you know my heart—I feel you answered in your own way—letting me discover the truth when I was ready."

My emotions raw, I consult close friends and several pastors. They all agree it's time to confront Ron. So many already have: Brian, then I, our professor; then the dean and another professor who was with him; and now it must be me again, with others. After much prayer, it's decided that Diane *and* her husband will be with me. I struggle, because deep inside I fear having to work on our marriage—I doubt I'll ever be able to trust Ron again. In prayer I admit, "I still want your will, and know I'll have your wisdom and strength for it, Lord. I pray Psalm 139:23–24 and Proverbs 3:5–8, 21–24."

Ron meets Diane and her husband, George, as we sit in my small living room where I've spent hours alone with God. He's with me now, I know. I plan to read from notes, since I fear I'll break down without them.

After reading Matthew 18:15–16, I say, "This is why Diane and George are here with me, Ron. I recently found out things that could've literally destroyed me had the Lord not been doing such a work in my life these past months."

I softly continue with the information Michael told me without divulging my source.

"I've been an incredible fool, but I don't regret it because I've been a fool who believed in you, and wanted to see and hope for the best. I've done all I can to put this marriage back together. I've asked your forgiveness and have a clear conscience."

I wait for what seems like forever for Ron to say something, but he remains silent with a stone face.

"I've lost all respect for you because of your self-pity, the flagrant defiling of our marriage contract and trust, the deception, the lies, the plan to divorce me and marry Jean, all while you tore down my personality and entire being with accusations and blame, to appease your conscience and justify your adultery. As it stands, there's no hope for reconciliation unless you repent and turn forever from this path with Jean."

Finally, Ron speaks, denying only one point, clarifying another in a way that only hurts more.

Then he says, "It was wrong. I wish I hadn't done it. I don't know why I did. Even when I didn't want to go back to her, I couldn't help myself. Anyway it's over. She doesn't want me anymore."

He looks like he's been tossed aside.

Diane asks, "Ron, am I hearing you say you feel worse that you lost Jean than sorry you were involved with her?"

"I'm hurting badly because I love her like I haven't loved Jo in years."

An arrow shoots straight into my heart, piercing it through. Then begins the blame, most of which I've heard, plus I'm a "religious fanatic," which is the reason Ron feels inferior to me. Diane and George just listen as I'm shriveling up. *He must be right.* I excuse myself to the bathroom where I cry out—"Help me, Lord."

I return, sit down and say, "I've been what you call 'legalistic' about marriage, believing God wants us to work this out. In these past few days I reached a point of not wanting to. Diane and George convinced me to be open. Ron, the easy thing would be to walk away. I believe we could *still work it out* with outside help, but decide soon. You've been involved with Jean nearly *two years*. I've tried to live up to your perfectionism and felt your unforgiveness so often. With all I have right now I forgive you, so you can have peace, which you don't have."

He says even that makes me "above him" spiritually.

After Diane and George leave, Ron stands at my door saying, "Can you *really* forgive me?"

"Yes."

"No matter what happens?"

"Yes."

I close the door and make my way to a chair, drawing my legs up under me.

The phone jars me out of my sobbing and hopeless pondering as Diane says, "We heard loud and clear all the blame he places on you and everyone but himself. Ron has no self-love, worth, acceptance, or forgiveness, so he must blame. We couldn't stand up for you because we felt Ron wouldn't open up if we did. I don't think he was repentant. He'd go back to Jean if she'd have him. It would take a miracle, but if he turns around, what a *ministry* you'll have. And if he doesn't, what a ministry you *already* have, Jo."

I cry as I hang up the phone.

You know how I feel, Lord. I don't want to be constantly put down by Ron for being who I am. I can't bear the thought of being married to him if he still loves Jean. I can't bear the thought of being fearful someone might see your light and hope shining through me because it intimidates Ron. But if he changes, I'll try—by your power.

In a few days Ron says, "I'm sorry for the way you found out about Jean. I think it destroyed our marriage."

I ask, "What are you saying?"

He answers, "I think we should proceed with the divorce. I'm sorry, Jo."

"I know. I hope you have peace some day."

"I hope you do, too."

I actually feel an odd relief after his phone call. In another way I'm numb. Numb to pain.

My voice always reveals exhaustion and stress, like now. I thank God for the Spirit's peace, presence and power; that I'm alive though I'll hurt, for I *can* trust God. Just days after Ron's decision, I ask God to use my voice as *his* instrument as I sing the solo "Yet, I Will Praise Him" with all three of the choirs backing me up. I shake with emotion afterwards, but I know it's true—I *do* praise God.

Chapter 7

Friends Care While I Grow

Anne and Dave, who have been dating, and other friends, eat hot fudge brownie sundaes with me in Hardees after the concert. Every song focused my heart on God, so my precarious future doesn't loom over me at the moment.

Anne says, grinning, "You ski great, paint well, *sing terrific.* Is there *anything* you can't do well?"

I answer, "Be a wife."

My friends disagree but *what do they really know?*

At ten the following evening a knock startles me. I spy Ron through the peephole and walk away, then feel supernatural strength dragging me back to open the door.

"I'm sorry to bother you, but I have something on my mind," Ron says.

I pause, wondering if I'll hear more blame, then motion to the couch.

His eyes pleading, he says, "I really wanted to tell you and make sure you know I meant I'm sorry for what I did. It was wrong, and I ask your forgiveness."

I answer tiredly, "I meant it last Tuesday night—I forgive you with all I can now—and that will grow. I want you to have peace."

"I didn't want you to know because I never wanted to hurt you. I can only imagine how much you hurt," he says.

"It's unbearable at times. I was such a fool, but I can be proud it was for the right reasons."

He says, "You believed in me. If I could only believe in myself. I just didn't grow, and I don't blame you for that. It wasn't your fault."

"What you're saying now is *so different* from last week when all I heard was blame," I say, confused.

"It's not your fault. You were a good wife and you loved me."

I sit crying, unable to grasp his words. "Thank you *so* much for telling me that."

Then he brings up the lawyers and I say, "I'll keep that in mind," and stand for Ron to leave.

Tears continue to trickle as I write—"TU *Lord.* I almost missed the opportunity for Ron to have more peace, and for him to tell me I was a *good wife.*"

I call Anne and she says, "You're like Ruffy—when she digs a hole, it's the best hole; when she wants to play, it's all-consuming. You're like that. When you ski, you give it your all, when you sing, you put your whole self into the song, when you paint … I knew you must have done that with your marriage—gave it your all and were a good wife."

"Oh Anne, thank you. Being compared to Ruffy is a compliment for sure!" and we laugh.

She adds, "You sounded soooo good at the concert, Jo."

All the affirmation I've received has inspired me to a concert ministry and our choir director, Ben, is anxious to set up a solo concert date at our church. I pray, "You care for me abundantly more than I can ask or *believe.* You *know* I love to sing for you."

Even though I'm on the honor roll, choir and especially madrigals top my list of classes in high school. I love the animated, a cappella singing back-and-forth around three sides of the table. Our music director recommends

I take private voice lessons, so Mom says she'll pay for them by wearing the same five outfits weekly—no new clothes. I feel really bad about that.

My voice teacher prepares me for scholarship tryouts with arias in French and Italian. The day I drive to Boulder, Colorado, I vocalize higher and higher on the curvy road. Then I notice the speedometer—*ninety miles per hour. I'd better quit vocalizing if this is how I drive!* I make the select madrigal group and qualify for a scholarship to the School of Music at the University of Colorado.

When our high school madrigal group performs in a supper club, guys wear black suits and girls long dresses with white brocade skirts. The pianist asks if anyone would like to sing a solo, so I raise my hand. He smiles with delight.

"What would you like to sing young lady?"

I ask, "Do you know, 'On a Clear Day'?"

He says, "I sure do," beginning the intro.

I start to croon, building the song gradually as if I'm a pro. Applause breaks out. It feels *so natural*. I'm a princess invited to her first ball—but best of all—*I've* been commissioned to sing the opening song.

I'm vocalizing when Ron calls about financial rearrangements, which I've been advised to leave with my lawyer. As Ron haggles I cry.

He says, "I wish I'd never done it. I was a jerk. It ruined our marriage."

I don't want to "take" Ron or make him uncomfortable, but all my doctors and PTs advise me *not* to work due to MS fatigue and debilitating attacks. "TU for being with me, Spirit. I panicked to think Ron might want to work on our relationship—how can I trust him? I don't know him any more. If you want me to try, somehow you'll empower me. You love me. I can trust *you*."

I awaken on June 21st and write—"Happy birthday, Jo—you are God's unrepeated miracle of creation. You love me so much! 'How precious to me are your thoughts, O God!'" (Psalm 139:17).

Anne, Dave and Ruffy take me camping the following weekend to celebrate. How I love these friends who listen to me pour out feelings of hurt and anger while I remember camping trips with Ron. I want the memories to end—they hurt *too much*. Jean's brother Brian called me a few days ago, saying, "Ron told Jean, 'It's God's will for us to be together.'"

At home I mutter through tears, "Jesus, You don't understand. Your spouse didn't have an affair! You were never married!" All of a sudden I realize God *does* understand. He— "… gave faithless Israel her certificate of divorce and sent her away because of all her adulteries" (Jeremiah 3:8). God *is* a divorced person! "Father God, I want to listen to you and know what part I play in your *grand scheme of things*. I want to live passionately, spending myself with love for others so that I feel alive even to my fingertips."

One afternoon as Mom helps me clean we tearfully discuss Dad. She's discouraged by his poor attitude. I'm glad I can listen. So often we don't mix—like oil and water. Mom tells me Dad wanted her to divorce him at one time!

She says she threatened, "If we get divorced, you'll *never* see your children again. I'm glad your dad and I didn't do that, we've shared lots of good times and he was a good father." I remember hearing after my grandfather left Grandmother he never saw my mother or aunt again.

It takes me three weeks to work up enough courage to walk to the pool using my new green crutches. As I lie on a lounge chair women ask about them, then MS.

One says, "It's so neat you can talk about it."

I slide into the pool frequently to cool off, explaining, "When I'm overheated, nerves can't conduct messages as well, so symptoms from areas of old inflammation show up."

I write later—"TU that I can walk with crutches and *not* be ashamed. TU for the confirmation that being honest about MS is *not* focusing on it too much."

Inga's letter arrives on a day when I sorely need encouragement:

"Jo, you are his loved daughter. You have so many gifts of him and he will use them through you. Christ and you are one. It is as you said: I am crying inside. We've prayed and hoped another way out. But we know you have done all you could. We pray for Ron that he should meet Jesus again and feel peace. Jo, we long for you. Will it be possible for you to come over here to see us again? We love you so much! Love, Inga and Ruben"

This evening my pianist and I are escorted through the prison gate to security where our things are searched on a steel table. After I share morsels about my life between songs, compassion covers prisoners' faces.

Later, Chaplain Morris says, "You can really relate to their feelings of hopelessness, being rejected, isolated, and alone. You have *such hope* to give others."

When I arrive home exhausted, I journal—"Oh God, you are my Lord and Savior. May your light shine through me (Philippians 2:15) and like Paul, through my weaknesses—when I'm with strangers or friends, in concerts or with MS counselees. Even when alone and only angels are watching."

The first counselee I speak with as a peer-counselor talks with such difficulty—halting and slurring—I can hardly understand her. When I get off the phone I pray, "Not my voice, Lord, *anything* but my voice." I'm crying as I consider not being able to tell people about God's love, to sing. Then I realize something else and pray, "*Everything I have is yours*—even my voice."

As I talk with a friend about feeling uncomfortable when asked what I "do" as in a job, she says, "Why? You have a great privilege of being an ambassador and minister of the Lord every day. Because of MS you can be used like no one else in so many varied and unique ways."

I pray, "Thanks for the *privilege,* as she put it so eloquently."

I'm excited to be asked to sing for the convocation of Denver Seminary, located in a nearby city. Then a friend recommends me to share the biblical perspective on suffering for a women's class there in the fall.

Ben calls, saying, "I think your voice is *better* because of the pain you've experienced."

Next I receive a letter from a friend at church near the seminary Ron and I used to attend. She writes she's instituting a choir award I inspired, "The Shining Star Award," based on Ephesians 5:13–14, and Luke 11:34–36. I write—"O God, you know I want to be a shining star for you."

But Ron files the divorce on June 28 and tears pour.

"God, you *know* I wanted to be a good wife. I tried so hard to please Ron. I wasn't perfect, but I loved him. The failure of marriage hurts. Ron's rejection hurts. I must remember you have something very special in mind for me."

Then he comes over, his eyes sunk in dark circles. He thinks he knows why "it" happened—he never felt he could open up to me about his feelings. I ask if he opened up to a friend or his family. I remind him how I supported and encouraged him.

"Men do that all the time—withhold their feelings, get frustrated, and think, 'Here's someone who'll listen to me' and have an affair. I tried to please you and you tore me to bits. *I felt like a nothing.*" Anger raises my voice, pain cracks it.

"You never really felt that way," Ron states.

I shoot back, "Want to bet? Ask Marsha, who scraped me up off the floor over the phone these past months at all hours so many times I can't remember. You nearly *destroyed* me as a person. I felt like a grain of sand ground under a boot."

As the conversation drags on for two hours I share my feelings in response to his continuing blame, ending with, "Brian asked me recently, 'What would you have *become* if your prayer to be what Ron wanted was *answered?*'"

At the door he says, "I'm sorry. I know you love me, and I've done so much wrong and caused so much hurt."

I call Diane who thinks Ron's still placing blame anywhere but on himself. Then I reread Christer's letter that came from Africa where he and Barbro are missionaries—"I am feeling so sad. I pray that Ron will find himself, a new self-esteem and a new dignity, and that he will come back to you. I pray that your love for him will remain, because I am sure that your life together is the will of God."

Can I trust you enough to keep my love for him? Will he ever change?

My neighbor, Jessica, joins me for stuffed acorn squash this evening. She nurses at a local hospital. I've learned her life has been painful, and until me she was wary of people who called themselves Christians.

Months ago she said, "Your husband was a *pastor*. Why don't you *turn* from God?"

I answered, "God is the *only* one I can really trust. Ron's making his own decisions. We have free choice whether to become Christians, and we continue to have it. If we weren't free, we wouldn't respond to God's love freely, which is what he wants."

A friend of Jessica's suggested before the divorce that *I* have an affair to make Ron jealous. I couldn't conceive of doing that. I knew it wouldn't please God and would only make me feel worse about myself. Besides, I only wanted Ron.

"Would you go with me to the singles' breakfast associated with my church, Jessica? I was scared at first, but now I love it."

She surprises me with, "Sure."

"There's something else I've been thinking about. I grew up camping every summer in Rocky Mountain National Park, then backpacked with Ron. I really would like to get into the backcountry by horse. Would you be interested?"

"Wow, that sounds like fun!" and we make plans for early August.

"Is this all of it?" the stable hand asks as he packs our one-burner stove in the top of the already full saddle pannier.

I gulp exaggeratedly, and answer, "Yep!" Suddenly, I look down at my forearm crutches and say, "You need to attach these."

Rowdy holds my horse's reins while I swing up into the saddle. *What in the world made Jessica agree to this harebrained scheme of mine—two women led into the backcountry by a cowboy we don't know who will ride out with our horses? And one of us has MS.*

I rode a few times growing up, and read recently horseback riding can actually *encourage* trunk coordination. I know with spasticity and nerve fiber pain due to MS, I could feel really bad, so I've continued leg raises with weights, hoping to curb at least saddle soreness. I used to feel I must be making up pain due to Dr. Black's opinion, now I know there are several kinds created by and related to MS.

Soon, we approach a swiftly moving creek.

"You won't have any trouble if you just keep urging your horse on with your feet. Keep control of the reins and he won't stop midstream. If he does, you might get wet!"

Great, nothing to it—keep control of a 1,000 pound animal who doesn't know me. Even though my feet touch water, which is obviously fairly deep, I must be fooling my horse for we don't stop. I pat his neck thankfully, saying, "Good boy."

Jessica yahoos when she reaches the bank.

Climbing higher on the rough and rocky path, a sprinkle glistens scenery I haven't relished for years. From 10,500 feet I spy trails I maneuvered in hiking boots before we descend 500 feet steeply into a gorge, sunlight shimmering on Odessa Lake, and we amble toward our wilderness site.

"Are you ready to be left alone up here?" Rowdy asks with his crooked smile still hanging lopsidedly on his ragged, whiskered face.

"Sure," I answer.

"Okay. See you in a few days. You take care now," he drawls as he hauls his muscular body up onto his horse and tips his Stetson.

We collapse in our tent for a nap just as the typical afternoon shower falls. After our celebration dinner we pile our food into a plastic bag, tie it closed, and hoist it up into a tree just like the rangers instructed. When a sliver of golden moon lights the sky and our fire dies down, we take a pan and lid into the tent to ward off marauding bears, then slip into our sleeping bags as the sounds of the warbling creak and critters we can't name serenade us.

While the gorge fills with a golden haze, Jessica and I are scrambling eggs when a park ranger appears, saying, "I heard about you two staying up here alone. Hope you made out okay last night. Seen any bears?" he asks a bit too casually.

Jessica answers, "I wouldn't have *heard* a bear as hard as I slept."

"Well," he says, laughing, "You should be glad. The campers only a half-mile away did. They had to run a bear off. It's a good thing you tied your food up there."

I sigh, thinking *how exciting,* then shake my head at my foolishness.

We spend the next two days exploring the area. When my energy is spent, it's spent; and I lie down to rest, sometimes slipping off to sleep. During one such time we sprawl on boulders baked by the sun. Later, I sketch the lake scene before me. I didn't think I'd *ever* be here again. Tears fill my eyes as gratitude fills my heart. Suddenly a couple wearing backpacks approach.

"Hi," she says. "It's *incredible* up here."

I nod and he asks, "Do you mind my asking why you use crutches?"

"I have multiple sclerosis," and he responds, "And you *backpacked up here?*"

"No, but I did years ago. This time we rode in on horses and we're staying a few days."

He asks if they can take our picture for his friend. "He really needs to know life is not over now that he has MS. You're the proof!"

If you only knew.

When Rowdy comes clopping into our campsite, I don't want to leave, no matter how dirty I am. Stable hands appear out of every nook and cranny when we three ride up to the barn and dismount.

I ask, "What's going on?"

"They want to see the women I took into the backcountry to stay by themselves."

"How many women have done this?"

Rowdy answers, "None," with that grin beginning to form.

Jessica and I look at each other in shock. Our exhausted bodies unconsciously straighten up, expanding with pride. As Jessica drives us home we talk about another adventure we'd like to take next summer. I smile at God, eyes drooping.

Bonnie Robinson, the president's wife and accompanist for the seminary convocation smiles sweetly. She tells me she didn't know anything about me before I arrived at her house to practice.

She says, "You are so beautiful, and your crutches add a certain other beauty—a kind of vulnerability. You have a great ministry for the Lord, Jo."

She must mean inside beauty, Lord, I can trust her.

The afternoon of the convocation I slip on the turquoise sleeveless wrap I sewed and pray, "Lord, calm me. Sing through me. Touch hearts tonight."

After I get a sound check on the mike with Bonnie, I pick up the brochure sitting on my chair placed in line with others on the program. When I see *Mrs.* Jo _____, I say, "Bonnie, I'm no longer a Mrs."

"But Jo, you are. The divorce isn't final yet."

I sense her compassion as tears well in my eyes.

When I'm introduced I pick up my crutches and walk to the stool provided for me before the huge church bursting with people. I nod to Bonnie, and her fingers stroke the keys sensitively until I begin to sing "The Journey."[9] This isn't a magnificently charged praise song—it tells of a life that will require faith in God. When I hear the roar of applause after my voice bares my soul I'm choking with emotion, not nerves. I chose this song, which Bonnie approved, because I don't want the seminarians to take lightly preparing to serve the Lord. *They will be tested.* My heart contracts in pain while I fight tears. Bonnie calls later to see I made it home safely.

She gives me a hug over the phone, saying, "I love you Jo."

TU, though this will be one of many hurts, you are with me, using me. I love you Lord. You're truly working Psalm 40 out in my life—"I waited patiently for the Lord; he turned to me and heard my cry. He lifted me out of the slimy pit … he set my feet on a rock and gave me a firm place to stand. He put a new song in my mouth, a hymn of praise to our God. Many will see and fear and put their trust in the Lord. Blessed is the man who makes the Lord his trust … I proclaim righteousness in the great assembly; I do not seal my lips, as you know, O Lord … I speak of your faithfulness and salvation. I do not conceal your love and your truth from the great assembly" (verses 1–4, 9–10).

After we talk for a while the next afternoon, a guy I meet at the pool tells me he'd like to call. *What does Carl see in me?* I ask many Christian friends about my seeing him and their opinions vary from "Don't date until the divorce is final" to "You're close to God, listening to his heart, I trust your decision." Carl drives me to the mountains. We laugh. Two men at singles' talk about me becoming strong enough to not need crutches—Carl accepts them as part of me, walking proudly nearby because I'm an "overcomer." I hear Carl's growth in his faith during our conversations and I'm excited to be Christ's light, feeling a great responsibility as well.

As I sit on the floor, years of scrapbooks lay stacked on the coffee table before me. Memories of one year of dating and fourteen years of marriage have been lovingly applied. Not the fifteenth. I throw away each page, keeping only a letter Ron wrote to his sister explaining why he was going to seminary so *he* can see how he felt—I couldn't have coerced him without drugs or hypnosis. I read what he wrote in Christmas and Valentine cards through the years before I had MS and think he really did love me in some way. I write—"The blame after I got MS was both of ours," and in bold letters—*Growth*

Anne and Dave are *engaged* and I'm thrilled, but they can't understand Carl's retreat. They think he should be supporting me. Then I read in *Suddenly Single*[10] *why* one shouldn't date until the divorce is over. I'm *dealing* with pain and loss when I could be glossing it over with fun, rescued by Carl out of growth God has for me. I thank God for my aloneness pushing me towards healing.

A knock on my door reveals Jessica.

I hug her as she says, "When I see Christians do things like Ron I wonder why give my heart to Jesus if that's what happens?"

I say, "That's Ron's problem, between him and the Lord. I'm not responsible for him, but I am for myself. None of us—even Christians— are perfect. We sin, but can be forgiven. Why else would the Bible be full of warnings for Christians about sin? Satan wants us to fall, to lose our joy and victory and be bad witnesses to others—to keep non-Christians from wanting to believe. He works harder at tempting people in ministry to sin because it seems they should live more perfect lives."

"I'm afraid I can't live up to the commitment," Jessica says.

I respond, "*No one* can live up to God's perfection alone. The Holy Spirit lives in us, and as we remember we are God's, and want to live for him, the Spirit helps us make right choices. If we make mistakes, we can agree with God about them, claim the forgiveness we already have based on Jesus' death for us, and go on living an abundant life."

"I'm so glad you're my friend. I really learned a lot tonight. It's sad that some Christians don't associate with non-Christians."

"You're right. This was a *great* way to spend my evening—with a precious friend and my precious Lord."

I lie on the couch, writing—"You are my love, my life, my all. Without you I am nothing and alone. I didn't want my marriage dissolved, but I want to go on, just you and me, Lord, even without someone to share life with. *Growth*"

As the court date draws near and the attorneys still haven't agreed, I cry out for peace, fearing stress will worsen the MS. One night after my concert at the prison I express to the chaplain my concerns.

He asks, "Jo, have you ever sat down in a wheelchair with a box of Kleenex and given up?"

I answer, "No."

"Well, you're not going to now. God hasn't brought you through all this to go down the tube. Is anyone going with you to court?"

"Yes."

"Do you have anyone else behind you?"

"Yes, of course."

He tells me to name them one by one with their faces in my mind, then says, "Every one of them will be with you along with the Lord."

My strength increases daily. My family supports me and Grandmother says she prays for what's best and she knows I'll have it because I stay close to God. I tell her I will. A couple evenings later I sit at my table with boxes of slides, including ones from Israel. "God, you know what's in my mind and heart. I've been amputated from Ron's family except for his parents. Dividing these up as a gift for Ron can be another puzzle piece for me, though. I gave. I loved. I grew. I know myself better than ever. You *are* in control and using this together for my good." I list half a page of positives, ending with—"I'm not a victim. *Growth*"

After putting on black slacks, a sweater, and my maroon blazer, I read Psalm 37:1–2—"Delight yourself in the Lord and he will give you the desires of your heart. Commit your way to the Lord, trust in him and he will do this." *Be anxious for nothing, Jo* (Philippians 4:6).

Anne and I arrive at the courthouse and I see all my supporters in my mind. Ron looks vulnerable as he comes over.

I say, "If you don't mind, I'd like the Carl F. H. Henry book. It has special meaning."

He says, "Fine."

I tell him I went through all the slides and have some in Anne's car.

He says, "*Thanks.*"

My attorney arrives, saying, "They've agreed to everything."

Thank you, God. He, Anne, and I sit on one side of a large maple table, with Ron and his attorney facing us. The referee at one end asks Ron "for the record" some questions. My nerves overload. I shake and Anne grasps my arm.

She whispers, "You're okay. You can make it."

Ron is asked if the marriage is irrevocably broken and he answers, "Yes."

"Is there any chance for reconciliation?"

"No."

My breath catches as I hear the finality. Anne squeezes harder. Fifteen years are ended as we exit the stifling chamber that feels as dead as my marriage.

Ron says, "Thanks again for the slides. I didn't expect that."

"I wanted to do it for you." I extend my hand. "Thanks for being reasonable."

Tears fill his eyes. "I'm sorry for what I did. I wish I'd never done it."

"Thank you for saying that. You need to be able to in order to heal."

"I'm sorry I couldn't show how bad I felt about it before. I know some reasons why I did it, but it was wrong."

I respond, "I pray for you."

He says, "I do for you, too. I'm glad your health is doing so well."

"I'm grateful to God."

I'm yours, Lord. Do with me whatever you choose.

Chapter 8

An Unexpected, Full Life

"It's Thanksgiving. I praise you in the midst of all my difficulties 'costing' me everything I *think* I need and want as I yield to you as Lord of all. My heart is exactly where *you* want it—on you, not my problems." I write my Christmas letter as a way of being thankful:

> "One year ago I was in despair. I loved Ron and prayed constantly for the reuniting of our marriage … My desire to not be bitter for the divorce must be an active choice because I don't believe it should be an easy panacea. The label divorcee isn't a pleasant one … Remember Ron in your prayers …"

My letter continues with all the wonderful things happening to me, then I pray, "God, TU, I *am* doing so much better. *You* make life worthwhile. TU for the Rices telling me on Thanksgiving Eve 1972 about you dying for me, Jesus."

Three days later I pray, "Let your light shine through me this evening at my first solo concert so that others see your good works and glorify you" (Matthew 5:16). I begin nervously, but as I share bits of my story of God's faithfulness between songs, I feel increasingly at ease. The look on Bonnie's face as she hands me a bouquet brings tears to my eyes. Affirmation pours over me like sparkling cider, fizzing from all who are proud of me. In bed I play the evening over and over, like an amazing movie. Finally, I get up to journal—"TU Jesus. It was *so* much fun to share with people what *you've* given me, what *you've* done in my life."

I want to celebrate Christmas this year, so I invite singles to my "tree-decorating party." We're stringing popcorn and cranberries, laughing, when our singles' pastor Mark asks loudly if I've taken a personality test.

I answer, "The Taylor-Johnson."[11]

Mark says, "Let me guess, you're self-assured, gregarious, perceptive, intuitive."

My cheeks redden as I say, "I guess you're close."

After everyone leaves I journal:

Growth Affirmation Eighteen months ago I would've cringed in fear because Ron would be angry, and I would've thought there was something *wrong* with that description. Now I can say TU for making me like I am. "The Lord is good to those whose hope is in him; to the one who seeks him" (Lamentations 3:25–26).

On Christmas morning at my parents' I say, "I'm so grateful for my family and our love," and break into a sob, so Mom comes over to hug me.

After opening gifts, while the turkey roasts, we pile into vehicles and drive into the mountains to slide on inner tubes and saucers on the snow for our ritual. Then Dad's belligerent negativity and ugliness douses the laughter with what seems like scalding water, as if to melt the snow and halt the fun.

One day Mom knocks on my door in tears. Dad called her a *slut*. We know he has little blood flowing into his heart with so many clogged arteries that can't be repaired again, but that's no excuse. Yet I remember growing up hearing them both saying ugly things to each other. It reminds me of watching "On Golden Pond" the other night. I felt like the bandage on my heart was peeling back a little. I wanted to grow old with Ron—*why did it have to happen this way?*

Then I receive a letter from friends in ministry. They're displeased I wrote that Ron divorced me. *Was I wrong?* "Lord, teach me," I pray. My cheerful friend, Ruth Peters, calls and says, "You weren't malicious, but there will be hurt. People need to know the truth to pray effectively."

I'm grateful for her call. Petite, azure-eyed Ruth entered my life with a bear hug from behind after I sang "Yet, I Will Praise Him" with all the choirs, whispering, "I love you and want to be your friend." Her family of Ken, witty and down-to-earth, and three fun children—David, Nathan, Anna—seem to be "adopting" me.

I drive the short distance to Cocos restaurant on a cold Saturday morning where any moment a ski-buddy driving to WP is picking me up. A guy I've never seen before getting into the car next to mine asks me to go to Vail *with him* to ski.

"No thanks," I say, astounded by his forwardness, thinking *he must be hard up to ask me!*

Then two guys and a woman on the other side of me go by, but not before the cute driver smiles. Using my crutches, I walk inside to get warm. As the minutes pass, I call and find out my ride's gone. *Maybe she's forgotten me.* The three people I'd seen earlier are leaving as I hear myself saying, "Where are you going skiing?"

When they answer in unison, "Winter Park," I say, "My ride hasn't showed. Do you think I could go with you if I help with gas? I can't believe my audacity, but you seem nice, and I really want to get there for a lesson."

I enjoy myself in the front seat with Brian until they casually mention smoking pot and pass around Peppermint Schnapps. After they drop me off I pray silently *I asked you to protect me and shine through me. I can't believe I did this, Lord!*

Dave greets me with a warm hug, but he's troubled that I asked for a ride from strangers, especially with their drinking and talk about marijuana. He says, "You're *not* going home with them."

I'm grateful for his protectiveness, especially at day's end when we enter the boisterous bar as Dave says, "There's someone from the office Jo can ride back with, so you guys can take your time."

Brian's face falls. As we walk away Dave remarks, "Jo, there are all kinds of guys out there, but there's a right one for you."

"Thank you *so much* for caring about me, both you and Anne."

"Jo, we *love* you. You're important to us."

When Anne calls later she says, "Dave said, 'Jo needs to realize she's pretty and smaller than most guys, and there are going to be a lot of them after her—but *not* always nice ones.'" I just shake my head in disbelief—*me? Ha!*

The following day I collapse.

I'm crying, God—you know. MS exhausted me today, even with two rests. I don't want to lose ground and be unable to live alone. TU for showing me I can help others with MS. I'm humbled the director considers me her best peer-counselor. I know it's because of you in me. I had to learn a lesson this week—I cannot deny I have MS. I must take care of myself or I feel worse. I need to practice what I preach to counselees! *Growth.*

One morning I journal:

Ruth said, "You're an inspiration to me, Jo. I think your journal should be published to help others." Interestingly, my women's Bible study teacher has been telling me the same thing. Lord, is this why I have MS? Or one of many reasons? You choose the things foreign to what the world considers good to be useful to you, because you don't want anyone to boast before you—you want us to boast in you (1 Corinthians 1:27–29). "We have this treasure in jars of clay to show that all this all-surpassing power is from you, not from us" (2 Corinthians 4:7). I want to boast in you.

Yet with all my boasting in God, grief still pins me to the couch at times when happy memories dissolve into pools of sadness on the floor. Then Anne invites me to a Bridal Festival. I can't imagine being there, but I can't imagine letting my dear friend down either. I actually share her joy and put aside painful thoughts. Another *growth.* When Anne talks with me about wedding rings and it doesn't hurt me—*growth.* Then Anne *shows* me her engagement ring. She sparkles and glows like the diamond she wears. I'm so happy for her I could burst—*growth.*

The next day I sit curled in a corner of my couch with tears dripping off my face, "Lord, I hurt. I mourn the loss of my marriage and love I thought we shared. I need *your* love to wrap around me like a soft robe. Protect me from being in a painful one-sided relationship where I give and give and am rejected and not loved. Thank you for the pain and grief and needs you alone can meet."

God is my constant companion, but I'm glad he puts friends in my life. Jessica and I spend hours laughing, crying, and sharing deep thoughts with each other.

One evening she says, "The thing I *don't* have together is my relationship with God. I'm really growing in understanding what that's like, because you explain it *and* you live it. I've watched you. Your faith is real."

I can hardly contain my excitement, but I'm even more thrilled when Jessica says, "I woke up thinking real hard about not wanting to go backwards to the way I've lived, but I'm afraid to give up the controls to God. I know I need to make a decision."

Jessica's fearful God will ask her to become a missionary nurse in Africa, so I say, "Why not give yourself to the one who loves you and *won't* give you more than you can handle without him?"

I pray for her every time I awaken.

My phone's ring wakes me with Jessica saying, "Guess why I'm calling?"

"Your car won't start?"

"Jo-o. *I gave my life to Jesus this morning.*"

I yell, "Thank you, God!"

Jessica comes over for a hug, so I say, "We need to have a 'coming-in' party for you—coming into *the family of God*," and she grins happily.

Jeff and Marsha host my next concert where he now pastors. Afterwards, Marsha says, hugging me, "I wondered a year ago if you'd ever sing again."

I answer, "God *is* faithful to heal."

As more ministry opportunities dot my calendar, Ruth suggests I use background tapes, especially since she's spoken with Stonecroft Ministries' leadership about my speaking and singing. A couple weeks later a guy from the breakfast says he wants to contact recording studios regarding background tapes and demos. I'm overwhelmed by John Cero's desire to pay for this. The Peters want to help as well!

> I'm so glad to be your child, to have your perspective on life. TU for the reason to sing—you've given me spring in my heart. Keep me close through your Spirit. I desire to not only say I want what's best; I want to believe what's best. Live what's best.

But dating terrifies me. A man with raven black hair named Terry appears at the breakfast and as we talk I say, "The only reason I'd ever want another relationship would be to share life. Everything is so special—just to be alive. To see buds on trees or fix banana pancakes, to share God's beauty and fun times, as well as the bad."

He says, "You *emanate* a desire to grasp at life and get it all."

The following Sunday a broad shouldered guy sits across from me.

As Randy talks about skiing I say, "I ski. We should go. I use outriggers when I ski, also to walk with, so I need to have my skis carried by someone. If I fall, I need help getting up because my ski tips are hooked together, but I'm pretty good."

I can't *believe* myself! Anne and Dave and others at WP have certainly given me confidence.

When Randy takes me skiing we have a great day. Later that week his parents ask about MS and after answering I say, "I get a lot out of life because I realize how precious and unpredictable it is."

Later, I ponder Ron saying, "Your zest for living will always be a problem for me," and I feel so sad for him.

I can't glory in my marriage. I can only glory in you, which is what you want, Lord. Every thought leads into the next, growing in importance, like a snowball getting bigger as it rolls down a hill:

> Now that someone interesting is in my life I'm afraid of being dumped because of MS. I'm afraid no one will take the time to see who I am deep inside—there's so much more than disease. I cannot avoid this fear because to risk is the only way to discover how someone really feels. I can only avoid it by walling myself off from possible hurt behind a con-

crete barrier. I can't do that because I want a great relationship someday. Someone will have a lot to prove. I must accept this fear and insecurity will probably accompany interest I have in anyone until the very special someone comes along who proves his devotion, trustworthiness, and love. Insight: Isaiah 41:10—"So do not fear, for I am with you; do not be dismayed, for I am your God. I will strengthen you and help you; I will uphold you with my righteous right hand."

Randy *likes* my love of life and God. He thinks my being strong is good. He isn't jealous or intimidated because I'm out-going. He compliments my skiing to others. We escape to the mountains; camp with others; and with me riding on the back of Terry's tandem bicycle, a group of us ride the trail over Vail Pass. I laugh and puff and pant and scream when we go downhill. I'm having *so much fun in life*.

A friend from choir hosting a tall, slim Norwegian tells him I ski well, and we decide to go to WP. Lars offers to be my host in Oslo, Norway, and with his friend who lives in Bergen, my prayerful plans to go to Sweden with money from Grandma's estate expand.

Summer nears but I have so much to do *before* then. John Cero set up a date in Denver since the studio producer who recorded backgrounds suggested I should be recording—and John wants to finance it! Though Ben wasn't surprised, I couldn't believe it. And my PT, Angela, tells me I must cut back one third of my activities—my rippling arm muscles indicate I'm overworked.

This evening I give my first concert singing to background tapes. The church is full with people I've never met, plus a few from hydrotherapy and the MS Society, singles, some family, and friends.

I say, "I'm grateful for my friends' support of activities I love doing, but I think it's important for *all* of us to remember Paul's verses in 2 Corinthians 4:16–18:

'Therefore we do not lose heart. Though outwardly we are wasting away, yet inwardly we are being renewed day by day. For our light and momentary troubles are achieving for us an eternal glory that far outweighs them all. So we fix our eyes not on what is seen, but on what is unseen. For what is seen is temporary, but what is unseen is eternal.'"

I look out into a sea of faces with eyes sparkling tearfully.

When I finish a woman in a flowery dress says, "I'm in a quartet and we give concerts, but *you minister.* Thank you so much."

A man using a cane says, "Thank you for talking about MS," and I squeeze him.

Later, as singles crowd around a long table at Cocos, seating me in the center, they tell me the verses really hit home.

The cyst grew from nothing, but its tiny presence in my hand at the joint of my second finger expands until it hurts to use my crutches or turn my steering wheel. I'm afraid of anesthesia triggering the MS. I've tried so hard to be independent. I'm afraid I'll face rejection from Randy and others who have seen me so strong, courageous, and able. I'll be too vulnerable, tender, needy. I feel like crying.

"Make me more like you through this surgery, Father."

Though I tell him my concern, the doctor will remove the cyst under a local anesthesia to which I've had a strange reaction before. I lie awake on the operating table with a band around my right arm while they remove the benign growth.

Then the anesthesiologist says, "We're going to release the arm block now and let the xylocaine into your system where it will gradually dissipate."

I can't hear anything. Where am I? Floating. Floating away.

"Jo, *wake up now.* Come on. Come on back."

I sense the oxygen mask over my mouth and nose. I blink my eyes. I can't move. I can't move *anything* except my eyes and mouth. Tears flow down the sides of my face into my hair and I can't wipe them. A green-clad nurse removes the mask and I look into a sea of concerned faces.

"I—I can't move."

I hear whispers as they consult one another. Eventually a nurse rolls me into Recovery, but I'm not recovering. *So this is what it feels like to be paralyzed. Maybe this is how Joni feels.* I pray silently, *Father, I'm afraid. I need your peace. I ask you to heal me though I know you can use me even if I remain paralyzed.* I pray this many times over the hours that pass until finally I can move a shoulder, an arm, my fingers, my legs.

When Mom's allowed to see me she says tearfully, "I was *so* worried."

My closest friends are surprised to hear how serious the surgery became, wishing they'd been there to help.

"I didn't want attention. I've been told I try to get it with illnesses."

Then Ron *himself* calls to give me his new address in the Midwest where he's relocated, and when he asks how I am, *he* voices concern and hopes I heal quickly. I journal—"Lord, it didn't hurt. It just seemed odd to talk honestly about health problems with him. *Growth*"

After Jessica drives me to the area-wide Stonecroft Ministries convention, I sing a solo then we head up to Buena Vista, the site of the singles' retreat. While attending a small group I find myself pouring out vulnerably how I've been feeling. After that, others spill their own emotions.

When we discuss "identity" I say, "I'm learning to answer the question 'What do you do?' with, 'I am growing in becoming more Christ-like. I give myself away through my MS peer-counseling and ministry.' I have a unique and interesting life and I'm happy." Once again I see tears in eyes surrounding me.

Following choir practice the following Wednesday, I say, "One year ago my world fell apart and I sang with all of you, 'Yet, I Will Praise Him.' I could do that because of your prayers. Now I've made it through this year and I can honestly sing this special, 'You Are There,' not only with you, but *to* God, and tell him you *have* been there for me."

Afterwards I say to Ben, "This has been the best year of my life—in spite of horrendous fear and hurt and rejection—because I've *known* God's love so powerfully, so abundantly, so sufficiently."

He says, "Jo, we can all see that in you."

For my birthday Anne and Dave as well as the Peters give me teddy bears. Now I have something to hold tight in bed, and to rest my shoulder on if it's sore. I'm so overwhelmed by the poem Ruth writes in their card, I ask Ben to read it with me:

"To You, Jo"

As we look into your face we see the beauty of our King.
As you bravely run your race, and as you live and love and sing,
You exalt His Holy Name, leaving none of us the same!
Happy Birthday, We love you, Jo, Ken and Ruth

Ben says, "It's true, Jo, that's who you are. You leave none of us the same. You've touched us all."

Tears well in my eyes as I say, "Tell me if you see me stumble or become someone I'm not because of wonderful things happening in my life. I'm overwhelmed by so much good."

Ben says, "Jo, you need a lot of good after all the bad. Just keep close to God."

I pray silently, *The need to be who I am in you is most important, not to any other person. TU for friends' affirmations, but you are my truth—you set me free to be me, Lord.*

I choose only songs for my first recording that hold deep meaning. John and Jessica pick a cover photo of me standing, using my crutches, on Vail Pass with Copper Mountain ski area in the background. "That's you, Jo, your essence." Friends sit with me throwing around names for the ministry and one of the songs I love to sing says it all, "His Music." So HIS MUSIC, Ltd. is born.

Then, only days before I fly overseas I write—"Today is R-day! I claim Psalm 25:1–3—"To you, O Lord, I lift up my soul; in you I trust, O my God … No one whose hope is in you will ever be put to shame.' I can't do this alone. MS would make me too fatigued. In my weakness be strong, Lord."

In the evening, as my mind and body feel like mush, I journal:

Oh God—you were magnificent. TU so much for Ruth's love, her precious accountability I need, her belief in me and criticism because she knows what I can do with my voice. TU for John's desire and ability to pay for the recording and believing in this ministry. TU for my life. To be honest—I can't understand it. I feel as if all the good might disappear in an instant with no warning. Why do you want to bless me this much?

Chapter 9

God Does Love Me This Much!

On the first leg of my journey I'm transfixed in a stupor. I can't grasp all the good. It's just too much. Landing at JFK, I wobble, but somehow find my jet leaving for Frankfurt. On the overseas flight I can't help sharing what God is doing in my life with the young Texan beside me.

I look around Baggage for the train that will take me to Frankfurt Station. I've read it's easy. It's not. A man staring through wire-rimmed glasses waves me toward a door. He grabs my suitcase on wheels and lifts it onto the train. Then he grabs *my arm* and pulls me onboard. *What is he going to do with me? Help, Lord.* As the train slows the man motions, picks up my suitcase, and motions again. I couldn't fight him for it if I wanted to. I follow in a daze as he leads me to suitcase-size lockers. He reaches for my ticket, points in the direction I must go, then disappears before I can thank him. *I know Hebrews 13:2 says strangers may be angels. God, was he sent by you?*

Later, a young man lifts my bag and we enter a cabin occupied by two teenagers where I collapse on the lower bunk. Totally unaccustomed to sleeping before others, I whisper, "God, protect me," and *amazingly,* fall soundly asleep.

Hours later we rumble into Stockholm. Inga and Ruben greet me with hugs and tears and shock—two years ago I used a wheelchair. Christer and Barbro, on missionary furlough, arrive and we all reminisce with wet eyes while we thank God for how he's taken such grief and used it for my good, then we pray for Ron.

At Solskinet, Inga and Ruben's two hundred-year-old summer home, I sojourn in Inga's loom house, where she usually weaves. Gratitude fills pages. We row a boat and swim, laughing gaily. I sit in an old armchair near a spinning wheel to begin needlepoint under Inga's tutelage. The traditional triangular Swedish pine hutch graces a corner of the room. I feel transported back into another time, relaxing in God's love poured into me through these friends.

Singing to my newly recorded backgrounds, I spill forth God's work, Klas translating sentence-by-sentence for me in the church he now pastors. I feel such compassion from Eva and Klas, who once wrote proudly about Ron and me as examples of a good marriage.

As Inga and Ruben later deliver me to the station, we roar with pleasure when we spot a moose on the hillside, so numerous in Sweden that moose crossing signs dot roadways. After tearful goodbyes, my train heads northeast where long-haired, guitar-playing Oddvar, and his shy, sweet wife, Rita live.

They watch me, aghast, as I get off the train with help and pull my suitcase, one crutch resting on top.

"You are *so strong!*" Oddvar exclaims.

I say, "In God I am."

I explain God's profound healing and again, feel only God's grace covering me like a soft down comforter. Oddvar, also a pastor, arranged for me to sing and speak in churches. Then we take excursions before I board another train that whisks me across northern Sweden's mountains into Norway, to the coastal town of Narvik. As I sway to the rhythm of the train, I recount my incredible journey and how I *know* God is with me to a young German. I give him a booklet like the Rices gave me in 1972 and pray for him.

When we arrive at Narvik he places my suitcase on the ground. By now I *know* I'm an oddball—*everyone* uses a backpack. I've booked passage on a coastal steamer, which departs from the Lofotens archipelago above the Arctic Circle, but first I must get to the dock *before* the hydrofoil leaves. *Ahhhh*, I breathe as I fall onto a seat while the boat skims the North Sea's surface. Looking back, striking mountains and clouds reflected in wavy patterns on the sea elicit, "Praise God," but when I step on the dock at Svolvaer, I *gasp*. Mountainous islands jut out of the North Sea, and the midnight sun, having never set, lights up towering peaks brilliantly with its ginger hue, giving glory to God, as if to say, "*Behold, he created everything. Enjoy it. Never forget he is God.*"

As I head uphill toward a hostel, young trekkers offer to carry my bag and I can't thank them enough. After resting I stroll along streets then sit in a pew in an old church and pray to take in how loved I am by God. My heart surges with gratitude that he's giving me strength to take this trip *alone*. Walking back, a man with a seductive look riding a bicycle haphazardly veers toward me and suddenly an elderly couple appears between us.

In broken English she says, "He show himself to women alone. We walk with you."

I say, "Thank you so much."

When we cross a street they disappear along with the odd man. *Were they, too, angels sent to protect me, Father? You are so good.*

A Swiss teacher carries my bag as I board the coastal steamer, and find my tiny cabin. The ship stops at each island with clouds folding over the tops of peaks like puffs of fake snow, the midnight sun rim-lighting them, and the sea rolls. I hang on while writing my feelings as a mist covers me. Then I literally bang from side-to-side of the corridor on the choppy sea. I'm glad I purchased Dramamine.

All along Norway's amazing coastline I bask in God's love. When the steamer reaches Bergen, a blond beauty walks up the gangplank, asking, "Are you Jo?"

I smile, saying, "Yes, are you Gerta Alice?"

She shows me the astounding view of Bergen, and when we visit the composer Edward Grieg's home, I look at the fjord from his cabin in the pines thinking *I could compose here, too.* Then I board the train bound for Oslo to visit Lars and his family. When I travel through the glacier-capped vaulting peaks to Malmo, Sweden, I can't stop grinning. I'm overflowing with God's love and joy.

Strangers assist me to the luxury liner bound for Harwich, England. Inga worried so about me being alone in London at a hostel, she called a friend who knew a pastor. He picks me up at the ship dock. I now *know* God holds me safely in his loving hands. I planned my trip carefully, but without help I wouldn't have made it, and I could've been taken advantage of *so often.* The Asian pastor takes me to his parishioner, Olive, who will be "me English mum," and I sing and speak in their church. I take the underground and trains, arriving at day's end at Olive's, barely walking. She fixes Ovalteen and draws me a bath. I'm warmed from the inside out, lit up by Olive's smile and God's care.

I return home having begun to *believe* deep in my soul God loves me so much he *wants* to bless me. I feel more "rooted" in God's love to *claim* the power to "grasp how wide and long and high and deep is the love of Christ" that he wants me to *experience*—even though its vastness is beyond comprehension—so that *he* will fill me (Ephesians 3:18–19).

When Mom arrives at the gate, she says, "I have a wheelchair."

I say, "Thanks, but I haven't used one for five weeks, *I won't now.*"

As soon as she drops me off, my phone rings.

"Hi Jo," Ron says, startling me. "I've been trying to get you for *a month.*"

"I've been away. I went to Sweden, Norway and England, on money from Grandma's estate."

He answers, "That's *great.*"

"I went by myself," wondering what that will mean to Ron.

"I'm sure that made you feel good."

I raise my eyebrows in surprise, saying, "It did."

"I've wanted to tell you all month how sorry I am for how I hurt you. I know I must have hurt you very badly, and I'm sorry for sounding callous, as if I didn't know you were hurt."

"Thank you for saying that. It *did* hurt badly. Although I tried, I had trouble believing God could use it together for my good, but I can now see he is."

"I never doubted it for you. You've always had a strong faith—stronger than mine. It's taken me a long time to say this, but I want to tell you I'm sorry I destroyed you so much, and I'm also sorry I destroyed our marriage."

"Me, too."

He continues, "I have a long way to go, but I'm learning. I tried to be something I wasn't for too long and cracked. It happens to a lot of people in ministry."

"Well, I'm glad you could say this, for me, *and* you. It will help you heal."

I soon say, "G'bye," and sprawl on my bed, journaling—"TU for the dream about Ron recently that prepared me for his call. Lord, he's still comparing himself to me. Still talks with low self-esteem. How can we *ever* make it work? He didn't even hint at it. You know I *would* try if you want me to, Lord."

Dating Randy fills my life with recreation as we camp with others and raft down the Arkansas River. I paddle until my arms give out, and wearing out one part of my body wears it all out due to MS. I'm so exhausted I need Randy's support to walk. I've overdone and will pay for it. *Oh, but it was a blast.*

Between our great times, my journal pages fill with concerns about Randy's frequent job changes, all too similar to Dad. Other things make me insecure, even after seven months. I carry a weight heavier than I used to haul backpacking. "Lord, show me what to do."

Mom told me when I invited Randy to a family barbecue months before, "I'm going to give Randy a big hug for putting up with all your faults."

I asked, "What do you mean?"

She answered, "Oh, you know, your MS." After meeting him she said, "Don't mess this up with things you say."

Both Marli and Mom told me to keep my mouth shut, just wait and see what develops. I realized their MO revolves around indirect communication, and now that I speak directly Mom feels I'll ruin this relationship, and my family wants me in one. I also realize this is part of Mom's *control.*

I'm a senior in high school dating a wrestler who also sings in madrigals. Mom seems fine with Sean. At the neighborhood Walgreens, an older brother of a friend begins to frequent my checkout counters. Finds me in aisles where I am stocking shelves. Says, "Bye" when I get off work as he hangs around outside.

When Steve finally asks me out he says, "Sorry my car's in the shop. I'll have to borrow my dad's."

I say, "That's okay," not realizing or caring that Steve is *known* for his Corvette Stingray. Steve is 21 and working full-time.

As December 31 nears, Mom tells me one evening, "Sean called to see if you were busy New Year's Eve and I said, 'No.'"

I look at her with tight lips, fuming. "You had *no* right to say that. I have a date with Steve."

Mom retorts, "You'll just have to tell Steve you forgot you already had plans to go with Sean."

I come home past curfew in the early morning New Year's Day and I'm grounded. And Mom thinks I'm safer with Sean.

Anne and Dave stand together, a beautiful couple I love dearly, saying their wedding vows. After singing "Never My Love," I lie in bed later singing songs Ron and I performed at weddings. I feel so cynical. Then I remember a guy from the breakfast saying, "Do *not* stop reaching out, Jo, it's what makes you, *you.*"

After Anne's wedding in Pennsylvania, with fall colors bursting just as she hoped and prayed, I visit with Kirsten and Jan Olov Stromberg, on sabbatical leave from a university in Norway, and a visiting professorship at Princeton. Ron and I stayed with them in Sweden in 1977.

Kerstin says, "God gave you a strong will and constitution, Jo. A strong mind. You bubble forth like a brook. That's what attracts men to you. You're an inspiration to me for how you want to go on to live, to rejoice, to grow, to exercise, to live the good life with God first."

Tears pool in my eyes as I hug her and say, "Thank you. I pray God will shine through me."

Jan Olov says, "He does."

When I return home I try to make sense of my anger at Ron for leaving me so fearful of trusting another. I call Ruth and say, "God's been working Romans 8:28 in my life—using me, releasing me to give him glory because of his love and power to heal and bring me joy. So I should be thankful, not angry."

She cautiously suggests, "Perhaps you're angry at God?"

"Not consciously, that's for sure. When Mark asked if I'd ever thought of turning against God I said, '*Never.*'"

Ruth says, "When we're angry at another person and let it fester, we're actually angry at God because he's in ultimate control. He knew Ron would do what he did."

"That's true. Though I don't think God desired it, he did allow it, and can use it for my good by changing me. I'm his clay. He's the potter. He wants to ultimately teach me to trust *him* first, then trust in others' love. 'I ask you, God, to forgive my anger at Ron and even you.'"

I feel a release in my heart, as if a prison door has been thrust open. "Thank you for forgiving my lack of trust in your sovereign plan to make me more Christ-like."

Ruth says, "Jo, you have an *inhuman* ability to trust. It's a God-given gift."

After we each say, "I love you," we hang up and I write—"PTL! *Growth and healing.*"

I'm thrilled to hear from Marilyn one evening. When I tell her about Ron's call she says, "It would never work for you two. You're way ahead of him spiritually *and* emotionally, and eventually he'd turn on you with jealousy about your ministry."

This fresh understanding helps me evaluate Randy—a great guy and loads of fun, but not the one for me. I've heard Joni has married Ken Tada after fearing there couldn't be someone strong enough emotionally and spiritually for her. I draw hope from that.

When I visit with Marsha and Jeff we discuss how anyone I date needs to come to the point of dealing with possible progression of MS.

Jeff affirms what I already know, "Anyone who marries you, Jo, will have to be ordained by God to do so."

Then I tell Mom it's over with Randy.

She says, "You don't always need to speak the truth even if you think it is truth. You have a problem with that. People won't change that much anyway, and what you say won't change them."

"I disagree. I've talked to counselors who said I should let my needs be known."

Mom pronounces, "I won't say anything *ever* again," trying to manipulate me with guilt.

I call Susie, a psychologist. "Your family increases your confusion, Jo, with their, 'Let it lie. Give him time to work through it,' kind of talk. Relationships need open communication."

My neurologist says my poor coordination—ataxia—is worse. My right ear sounds like a flag flapping in the wind. If I don't get better within a week of resting she wants me to take prednisone. At Bible study I share how frightened I was to barely walk across my living room and a friend puts his arm around me, saying, "You really do live with this *every* day, don't you? We need to pray for you more."

I think about my trip last summer and *know* it was miraculous. I could *not* have done it without God's strength.

Since there isn't a stool for me during the choir Christmas program, Cindy puts her arm around me. As I weaken, I rely more and more on her. My humiliation grows. I fight tears. Suddenly I think of Tammy's words, "Remember, you're an example to the audience. Many with disabilities would just stay home, including my mom who has MS." From a stool delivered later, I sing my solo in the Spirit's power, mine long-since used up.

> I realize I prayed before the concert you would be glorified and shine through me *no matter what*. You showed in my weakness you *are* strong. TU Jesus. I also need to remember it's *my pride* that doesn't want me to look weak or fail, and that is *not* Christ-likeness, for sure.

I want to feel close to my family at Rhonda's for Christmas, but each time I talk about my life or express an opinion I feel cut off. I ask God if it's just my "over-sensitivity" I heard growing up, but as I journal conversations I believe I'm right.

A family member who's an occupational therapist (OT) says we shouldn't accept limitations for Dad.

I say, "As an MS peer-counselor, I disagree. Sometimes we must."

Another family member says, "I think he has lots more experience counseling than *you*, Jo."

I silently pray for God's light to shine down truth and for God to show me *his* outlook. During a hike the next day, when I can no longer walk due to muscle fatigue and resulting pain, I say, "I have limitations. If I ignore them I'll need your help more than either you *or* I want."

Dad stubbornly refuses to go to the Christmas Eve service. He demeans Mom in front of others at a ballgame, putting her in tears. Back at Rhonda's, Mom finds Dad on the bathroom floor. A sibling believes he's had a small stroke. As we all discuss Mom's situation with Dad, stress builds and harsh words volley back and forth.

When one says, "Mom should just leave Dad alone for a few days so he appreciates her more," because I know it isn't only Dad who can be mean, I say, "I don't want Mom to feel guilty after Dad's gone."

I kiss Rhonda and Tim goodbye before I step into my folks' motor home. After I help Mom get Grandmother and Dad ready for bed, then up the next morning, I pray, "I must take care of myself. I don't want to become dependent on others. Teach me to be loving—true love is shown through the rough times. Patience isn't learned unless there must be waiting, perhaps wondering. TU for this opportunity to prove and test me."

The next day Dad calls Mom a wench, meant as a sexual insult.

I state, "I'm not going to listen to this."

He says, "You're *just* like her, *a wench*."

"Yes, I'm like her. I have good and bad from *both* of you. I love you."

I drive home crying, wondering why Dad is so mean.

During our next HIS MUSIC meeting John talks about the ministry like a pregnant father. I must make him understand I *can't* handle a schedule traveling with one-night-stands. I'm grateful when each person takes on a responsibility to make the ministry possible. Clay, a widower from singles', wants to volunteer as well.

He says, "Your most shining attribute Jo, is your love for the Lord and desire to do his will. Your transparency is wonderful."

John, Ruth, *and* Clay want to trade off running our professional sound equipment. I journal—"I want this ministry to grow according to *your* will. TU so much for my friends."

After a concert where my mind fights not to impress Judie Amen, the women's ministry director for Galilee Baptist, and the Spirit wins by taking over, she says, "You *must* have an hour for our spring luncheon. Your simplistic faith—he's my God. Your total performance came across selfless, with integrity and authenticity as you share your life, not just singing, with the Holy Spirit working through you."

Oh God, you *know* I want to be like Judie said. My life will never be boring if you're always at work to make me like Jesus. My life will always reveal love and faith if I'm growing in you—*keep me growing forever*—even through pain!

Then I minister to women from many churches. Bonnie's delighted to hear my vulnerability, saying, "That's what vulnerability means, Jo, to risk being hurt."

Lee McDowell, a pastor's wife, says, "The most blessed among women was told she would suffer, Jo. To be a Christian is to suffer."

I ride home thinking *how true, Lord.*

When John discovers the only way to have my recording played over the radio is to have a record pressed, Anne and Dave donate towards the expense. So do Clay and John. I can't stop crying, I feel so blessed. It's more than I ever dreamed would happen to me—simple Jo.

In January I drive to the YMCA Camp outside the town of Estes Park near Rocky Mountain National Park to enjoy three nights at Clay's expense. *I dedicate this to you, Lord. Write songs through me. I'll rejoice in your beauty. Keep me safe.* I'm so exhausted I have chills up and down my spine. It's happened before after skiing. My back muscles spasm so I pile quilts over me. Then I awaken to a blanket of freshly fallen snow covering the peaks and draping the pines I love. I pull on jeans and a parka over my wool sweater and wander outside.

Words and a melody flow so quickly I hurry inside to jot them down and sing into a tape recorder to add to those begun on the steamer, now the song, "My Heart Wants to Cry Out, Lord!" As I ponder God's incredible power to heal emotionally, I write (with Ruth later helping by adding a couple lines that make the last chorus work):

"You've Brought Me Through Heartache … to Soaring on Broken Wings"

Last night as I sat pondering in my cabin in the pines,
I thought where you have brought me in the last few years of time.
You've brought me, Lord, to know your comfort, your ever-faithful care,
To learn to trust in you alone because you're always there.
You've brought me through heartache, through the hurt, the pain, the fear,
From the praying to go home to you, to knowing I can endure.
I can't help wondering, Lord, where I'd be, had I not known who you are
If I'd really been alone, without you—bitter, hopeless, hard.
I know I thank you for the good times—I thank you for much more
Thanks to you, Lord, for the tough times, for that's when I've learned to soar.
You've brought me through heartache, through the hurt the pain it brings,
From the praying to go home to you to soaring on broken wings.[12]

As I pray about relationships and think about Ron a song pours from my heart one night:

"He Knows"

When you stand beside your loved one—hurting, down in pain,
Do you ever wonder where God is, has he turned away in shame?
And has he left his child to take all the blame?
Does anger build up deep inside you at the One who could change the course
Of disease and illness, suffering, heartache—the One who is our source?
He knows your hurt, your fear, he knows your suffering.
He's always there with you, but his sovereign will is true.
Do you find you cannot praise him as you know the Bible teaches?
Thanks for good things isn't possible, your despair has endless reaches—
Those Scripture words are only pretty speeches.
You're feeling almost stifled, giving up and running seems the way
To rid you of the hurt and anger—that's when I've got to say
He knows ... his sovereign will is true.
He has the power to heal, but sometimes allows the pain;
Building strength and faith in you—
So that you can show, too—his power is perfected in weaknesses.[13]

Back home I submit my testimony to Stonecroft Ministries for approval. I'm asked to clarify—Why did you feel in despair and the ugliest girl in school? Was it your parents' arguing?—I have no idea. I only know I wanted, sought, and *had* to please my parents, and when they argued, *I* failed *them*.

When a successful businessman I met back East comes to town, he invites me to dinner. Henry speaks with hopelessness about his wife's illness. As I share how I must keep hope he reaches across the table for my hand and strokes it.

I say, "Pray I keep my eyes on Jesus," and Henry asks me to pray he'll do the same.

As I read the words to my songs "He Knows" and "You've Brought Me Through Heartache," he tears up.

"Your wife must be very special. I'd love to meet her someday."

Henry says, "She *is*. I'll tell her about our evening."

Later we say goodnight warmly.

In the morning I tell Ruth, "You know, I think if I'd hungered, this could've been Satan's attempt to ruin many lives. I thank God for his perceptions when Henry took my hand, and for giving me words to encourage a hurting man. He said, 'Be bold and open and share as you do, Jo. People *will be helped* as I've been. The rejection and negative tapes you say play in your head are not comparable to how you can help others.'"

Those tapes play on because Ruth is working on a write-up, and I don't want to defame Ron. It takes the wisdom of many, including a seminary prof, for me to see I *am* being fair when I tell the truth, not vengeful. It doesn't mean I haven't forgiven Ron. Hiding the truth won't work (Proverbs 26:26). I finally see Ron has said he's sorry, but he hasn't been *reconciled* because he doesn't want to work on our marriage. And if he did, Ron would let God work in him, and I *would* be able to grow to trust and love him.

As I sing, Anne plays a new melody of mine on the old upright piano I now cherish. Clay and Ken and I drove up to Nederland in the mountains to pick it up.

The phone rings and I make my way holding onto furniture and walls to answer it.

"Hi, this is Ray Franz from the singles' breakfast."

I rack my brain to think of who he is among the hundred or so people and say, "I'm sorry, but I can't put your face with your name."

"I sat next to Jay yesterday and talked with you."

"Oh, sure. Don't feel badly, there are so many new faces and I'm terrible with names."

Ray says, "I was just wondering if you'd like to go out sometime and get to know me better."

I hesitate and answer, "That's a possibility. Could I call you back later? I have a friend here."

After Ray says, "Sure," and I jot down his number, I plop down next to Anne.

"A new guy from the breakfast asked me out." She shrugs. "You've been wondering if you should be dating others besides Brad."

"But I don't *know* this guy. You know how hard it's getting for me to go out with guys I don't know at least a little."

Anne says, laughing, "Well, you can't interview him first, Jo."

I come back with, "Yes I *can*."

Chapter 10

Surprise Interest with Additional Blessings

When Ray answers, I discover he likes bicycling, so I say, "I enjoy riding the back of a tandem."

He skis and I say, "I use special equipment, but I *love* to ski." He also hikes up 14,000-foot peaks.

"I used to backpack and hike long distances." I pause.

With a frown on my face I say, "Umm—you *do* know I have multiple sclerosis, don't you?"

He answers, "No, I didn't. I know a little bit about it because a friend's wife has MS. He's told me about her struggles, but she doesn't let it stop her from enjoying life."

"I'm glad. It keeps me from taking life for granted."

"That's *great*. I used to do that until a tragedy caused me to see what I have." Ray's voice softens. "It was my divorce. I've been raising my young daughters by myself since Lindsey was three and Melissia one, still in diapers. Everywhere I went I carried a diaper bag," Ray laughs and so do I.

"Melissia is almost seven and Lindsey's nine, so it's getting easier. All you can do is your best and trust them to God. I sure love them. I help direct the children's choir at church. I haven't done much with singles for a while and thought I'd begin again."

I remember now. Ray joined Jessica and me two weeks ago in the parking lot. His smile spread beneath his dark mustache and his hazel eyes twinkled down at us in the bright sunshine. And yesterday at the breakfast, when a few of us gals were wearing hats, I felt someone staring at me. I wore my pink dress and black felt hat Ruth told me I just had *to buy. I peeked through the net to see it was Ray.*

He says, "I *would* like to take you out sometime."

"You didn't know I have MS. I understand if you'd like to renege," but Ray reiterates his desire and we set up a date a week away.

April 28, 1986. Well, Lord, I don't know what you're up to, but I'm excited. I enjoyed the *interview!* He's secure in his job of many years. Has children he loves, and even knows Ruth since they go to the same church now. He'll probably date lots of women from the breakfast.

Then I call Jessica who states, "Last summer I played on the church softball team and girls ogled Ray. You should *definitely* go out with him." I'm tickled by her assessment.

The following week conversations with Brad lead me to wonder *why* I get wrapped up with men like him. I flip back through journal pages to an evaluation I made months ago—I need a man who admits he needs a woman's nurturing so he will *not* turn against me. He needs to be a Christian growing in his faith. And adventuresome, because Ken told Ruth he sees that as essential. He's right. I need a man who realizes I'd be adventuresome even if I need a wheelchair, or have to be carried!

On Friday, a week before our date, I'm practicing songs at Ruth's church as Ray walks straight towards me while a group of children appear. I notice his dark brown, almost black wavy hair above his high forehead. Full eyebrows complement his smiling eyes with long eyelashes. I extend my hand and he grips it firmly. When Ray introduces Lindsey and Melissia I think *they're so cute.* Melissia's smile reveals dimples in her round cheeks, and her crystal blue eyes light up. Both girls have honey-blonde hair with Lindsey's a tiny bit lighter. Her small face with caramel-colored eyes like her daddy's is framed with bangs and shoulder-length hair like Melissia's, and she has one dimple. Lindsey stands a few inches taller and is a tad thinner than her younger sister. They skip away to join the choir going on a retreat.

Ray says, "I'm looking forward to our date."

"So am I."

When I arrive home I write—"Seeing good-looking Ray tonight has me wondering *why me?* I think he's interested, but I don't get it. He has two darling daughters. Isn't he afraid taking me out is *dumb* since I have MS? I'm intrigued."

In a few days John delights me with a box of record albums. We hug happily. I pray, "Hallelujah! Lead radio stations to play it for your glory, honor and praise."

After John leaves I make a decision I've prayed over for weeks. I need a D&C to remove abnormal uterine cells, and I've decided to proceed with an orthopedic surgeon's suggestion to remove scar tissue from my left hand while I'm under anesthesia. About sixteen years ago two ganglion cysts were removed from my left wrist, and the subsequent scar tissue build-up causes my first finger to point straight out when I bend my wrist. Stiffness bothers me now, not vanity. Friends say I rub it without even knowing. I schedule the surgeries for two weeks away.

When Ray calls in the evening, he tells me he was devastated when his wife left, but he's learned he wasn't all he should've been as a husband. He tried for three years to win her back to their home, going to a counselor alone. He finally realized he needed to change for himself, whether or not she returned. *I realized the same thing.* He knows he's grown and holds no bitterness. He's in a house Bible study group and was in another group led by Hal and Peg. *Neat people I've heard about at church.* He admits to not being as close to God as he wants, though, because he's successful right now. *He sees this!* When we finally hang up I pray, "I feel giddy and excited. Lead us, Lord." My day began *and* ends in delight!

Ray arrives the following evening wearing navy slacks and a plaid sport shirt, grinning. I'm wearing my magenta sleeveless blouse tucked into trousers with sandals. As we discuss movies, he suggests the comedy *Short Circuit* at a drive-in. My mind zings back to all my high school dates at drive-ins who only wanted to make-out. I agree to it thinking, *Surely Ray is different,* grab my crutches, and walk to Ray's silver Mustang SVO where he opens the door for me.

We sit in his sporty car's bucket seats talking through the entire movie. The only thing I pick up is the robot's name—"Number Five." I'm turned in my seat with my left knee on the console as I tell Ray there aren't many men like him.

He says, "I usually scare people off."

I put my head back and laugh, "Not *me*. It's great to be so open."

When Ray tells me I have a really nice personality and am a beautiful woman inside and out, I feel shy and thank him. Then I tell him about Anne's teasing that I couldn't interview him first. We chuckle.

I say, "Seriously, I'm cautious. I've dated a few guys and never thought that would happen. I've learned a lot the hard way."

Ray responds in the popcorn-scented car, "I've learned I have to make things happen. I met you, thought you were a very nice and *very* attractive girl, and wanted to get to know you."

"You *really didn't know* I have MS?"

"No."

I scrunch my eyebrows together and say, "Why did you think I used crutches?"

Ray looks at me, shadows dancing on his face from the movie, "I didn't even notice them."

Incredulously, I ask, *"Even when we walked side-by-side?"*

Ray answers, "No."

I shake my head, turn away, and say, "Ron eventually said he was disgusted when I used the crutches or wheelchair. Lots of marriages MS hits end in divorce."

"My friend told me that."

I go on, "But marriages that begin with acceptance of MS or any disease have better-than-average odds because they know they're dealing with tough issues, and work at it."

Ray shares that he's ready to risk in a relationship, though he's afraid. He asks, "Do you turn down compliments?"

I think *well, ones about my looks I doubt,* but answer, "Not usually, though I still have to turn off negative tapes. I think I know who I am. I'm learning I don't want to rescue someone for years so I have to be careful, because I'm an encourager. Still, I realize *I* need some encouragement. When the MS is a little worse, I'm exhausted, or more off-balance, I don't feel as good about myself. It's common."

While we devour strawberry pie at Marie Callender's Restaurant, Ray asks, "Do you get depressed?"

I answer, "I wouldn't call it depression. If I don't feel good, my emotions rise to the surface and I cry easily. My close friends listen to how I feel and share my burden. It really helps."

"Those are *good friends.*"

Ray tells me though he gets down sometimes, he wants God to be first in his life and to know him better. I smile, biting my lower lip, agreeing with him wholeheartedly.

Back at my apartment I play a bit of my album. He says, "You have a nice voice. And you're proud of this?"

I think for a moment before answering, "Yes, though I know there are many errors."

I look up at this really good-looking man standing next to me and feel excitement tingle inside. Sparks seem to fly. I think Ray feels the chemistry as I touch his arm with mine to balance myself while I tell about the photos on the back.

Ray says, "I envy you because you can do this."

"Don't. You can manage people. I can sing."

"I don't always manage well."

Laughing, I say, "I can't always sing well."

Ray's ready to leave so I tilt my head and venture, "I'm a hugger. Is it alright if I give you a hug?"

He answers with a disarming smile, "Sure," and puts out his strong arms. My head goes to his chest as I think, *oh, a nice big hug*. I close the door and write:

Wow! I'm smitten! He made a great impression! He said he's sorry to not hear me sing Sunday, but I urged him to go ahead to the breakfast since he's missed it. He's *terrific*, Lord. I feel like a schoolgirl. How I hope he wants to take me out again! Really, though, I know friendship is most important. I do hope he calls me, but there are lots of great gals for him to compare me to-ha!

Following church where I sing solos, I drive Grandmother to Echo Lake for a picnic. Sun sparkles like glitter on the water. Grandmother's feeling perky. She's had a rough time, breaking her hip, feeling useless, unable to get to church easily. I had told her in the hospital while she looked tiny and frail and depressed, "Grandmother, remember, your greatest ministry is still prayer. You can do that anywhere."

She said, "Yes, you're right, Josie. You're so wonderful. You're the only one I can talk to this way."

I said, "You've always been an inspiration to me to keep going, push on, never give up, and still know there's more to learn about God at your age! Maybe now you're to learn to praise the Lord though you're not being able to get out much." Tears filled my eyes. "I realize I won't have you forever, but I know you'll be such a blessing to Jesus."

She smiled wistfully and said, "Won't it be grand when we're there together? Won't we have a glorious time!"

As I drive her home I ponder being with Jesus. What *will* it be like? Upon opening my door I hurry to answer the phone and hear Brad's voice. *I'm so frustrated for being involved with another man who reminds me of Dad.* I lean on my redwood deck rail realizing I just wish Ray would call. I'm drawn to my answering machine as if I'm being reeled in by a fishing pole, and when I push the button I hear Ray's voice asking me to call him back. *Well, he went to the breakfast and still wants to see me. Yeah!*

Ray's taking his girls to the mountains for breakfast and a hike on Friday and they want me to go along.

"I'd love to Ray, and tell the girls 'Thanks,' but I have a busy day. Can I have a rain check?"

Ray says, "Sure," then invites me to the children's concert, but I have my own to give.

Ray asks, "Are you going on the single's retreat?"

"No, I'm having surgery."

His voice fills with concern as he asks, "Really, what for?"

"You probably noticed my first finger on my left hand points straight out like a hunting dog spotting its prey?"

He snickers while I explain the rest of the surgery.

Ray says gently, "I had a really great time Friday."

I almost whisper, "Me, too. I've already written on a card to send you."

"I've been looking for just the right one, but I don't want to frighten you off!"

"Neither do *I.*"

When Ray tells me he's planning to take the girls to Ouray and Mesa Verde I say, "That's *great.* I love it over there."

We continue a long talk before he ends with, "I'll call you!" and I grin.

Two days later I throw a dinner party for fifteen unique friends who bless my life and HIS MUSIC with their variety of helps and gifts. Ben and his wife encouraged me these past years, and his prayer reflects my desire, "Use Jo for *your* glory, Lord."

The following morning I discover my car isn't worth the repair work it needs. When I call Ruth, concerned about how I'll make loan payments to my parents, she reminds me it's sin to worry (Matthew 6:25–34). I pray, "I ask your forgiveness for the sin of doubt and worry. TU for forgiving me. I trust you to work a miracle in my budget."

After the rewarding luncheon for MS volunteers, the emotional healing seminar in the evening opens my eyes to childhood difficulties in men I've dated, as well as Ron. I pray silently, *Lord, I want to see any patterns from my own childhood that have me bogged down. Or have I already seen them?*

Peg comes up to me, saying, "We know someone you're dating and we think it's great."

"Ray's a wonderful person. So open."

"I'm excited to hear he's opening up and risking. He's been afraid. He wants honesty, not game-playing."

"Oh, I totally agree." As she walks away I pray, *Guide me each step, Lord.*

The next evening in a Church of God, my chin trembles as I point one finger heavenward toward God in praise, fighting tears during the standing ovation after my concert. During conversations, I silently thank God for touching individuals in unique ways through what I said or sang.

The pastor says, "I want you to know I see the light of Jesus shining through you." Tears glaze my eyes as he continues, "And I want to give you a pearl of truth. In Romans 8:28 the Greek emphasis is not on *all* things, but on *God* who works all things for the good of those who love him."

"Thank you so much for showing me this."

He adds, "I pray you can sing to a crowd at Red Rocks Amphitheatre someday."

"I just want to go where God wants me, sir."

He nods with a smile as his wife takes hold of me so tightly my earring digs into my ear. Her face wet with tears presses against mine as she says, "I love you," while my tears meld with hers.

After John brings me home I pray, "God, I want to remain humbled and grateful to be your servant. I'm privileged, I guess, to be like Paul in 2 Corinthians 12:7–10—I boast in my weaknesses, for then I'm strong in you. I seek *pure* motives."

I'm startled from my prayer by the phone's ring.

"Hi Jo!" Ruth shouts with glee. I can see her grin. "How did the concert go?"

I answer, and though she's thrilled I sense her distraction. Then she says, "Ray called and said, 'Tell me about Jo!' He's not afraid of the MS. His friend's wife has it, and he thinks it just makes her stronger and more beautiful, an asset to the family. Ray thinks the same about you. This guy's serious! I told him, 'I've read Jo's journal. It's like a diary and she's very real.

There aren't many in the world like her.' Ray told me he knew that already. Hope you sleep well!"

I respond, laughing, "How *can* I now!" *I remember handing over my journal to Ruth hesitantly before flying overseas because she wanted to write about me.*

When Ray's card arrives it feels like I've unwrapped a gift—he wrote how very comfortable he feels sharing with me—the *same thing* I wrote. He signed it, "You're a very special person, and I hope we get the chance to get together again soon. Ray."

My smile lights up my living room with a warm glow.

Surgery tomorrow. Various fears bind me in chains. My peace shattered, I discover the cries within:

> Ron was with me except the last time. My debilitating self-talk is *I can't go it alone.* The *truth* is I *am* strong in you, Lord. I do *not* have to be afraid. I'm also uncomfortable staying with Mom and Dad. Since the doctor doesn't want me staying alone, I ask you to use me to grow Mom's acceptance of others. I want to be so Spirit-filled I'm a blessing and bring *you* glory.

Then God pumps me up with encouraging calls from friends, and even a card from Ron's parents. After surgery the specialist says he had to make a longer incision than expected, and not to be shocked. When I finally see the Z-shaped scar down the top of my wrist and hand, I joke about having "The Mark of Zorro." I'm glad I don't model my hands for a living.

Even with the nurse's help, I wobble uncontrollably. MS rages for attention and my doctors comply with steroids. Friends and family visit, then one evening I hear Ray's compassionate voice saying, "I've been calling your apartment since I got back in town, then finally called Ruth. I thought your surgery was *next* week. How *are* you?"

After answering I ask, "Would you like to come visit? I have a friend here but he'll be gone soon."

I sigh with relief when Brad leaves mere minutes before Ray, Lindsey and Melissia arrive. The girls look scared, but when I invite them up on the bed, we hug and it feels like we're having a party. Ray tells me they picked out the flower arrangement.

After staying at my parents' a couple days, Ray calls and I ask if he'd like to rescue me for a bite to eat.

He says, "Sure. I was going to ask if I could visit but wondered if you feel good enough."

After they meet my folks, the girls play "dress-up" with old clothes like I used to, modeling for us. Later, Ray supports my left arm since I can't use my crutch when we head to his car, with Lindsey teasing, "I bet you *can't wait* to get to the car to see what we've got for you!"

I laugh while thinking how easy it is to be supported by Ray. *He's such a dear man, Lord.* Lindsey reaches into the car grinning, then nestles into my arms a stuffed koala.

My mouth opens wide with joy as Ray says, "I searched through a number of stores for this."

We name her Katy Koala as we drive to Show Biz Pizza.

The girls begin telling me about their pre-school half-sister. Soon, Lindsey asks if I have children, and I answer, "No."

Melissia asks, "Did you want any?"

"Oh yes, but God didn't plan that for me."

Melissia turns her face up to me, her big blue eyes sincere, saying, "I wish you were our new mommy."

I see Ray's ruddy complexion deepening in hue, so I say, "That's wonderful, but you have a mommy, and I'm just really glad to be getting to know all of you. I enjoy you *so* much."

Then Lindsey asks if I wish I didn't get MS when I was a little girl, but I explain I was twenty-seven when symptoms began. All three begin peppering me with questions which I encourage. Ray asks how the doctors know which kind of MS I have.

I answer, "By watching it, but that doesn't always hold true. I have no guarantees."

Ray says, "None of us do."

As I ask Ray to help me to the restroom I say, "I hope my wobbliness doesn't embarrass you."

"Not at all."

Tenderly, the girls help me inside.

After hugs to all three, Ray walks me to my folks' front door, and as he lets go and I walk inside, it feels like that spark would ignite if we touched again. I write to each:

"Dear Ray, Thanks for the blessing of letting me get to know you three. Your daughters have obviously been given lots of love for them to have so much to give freely away. Their spirits are so sweet, forthright, and refreshing. I respect you a lot for what I see in them. I was *so* impressed with you bringing Melissia and Lindsey to the hospital. Thanks for … I look forward to seeing you Friday. With Christ's love, Jo"

"Dear Lindsey, Thank you for your lovely pictures of rainbows and happy thoughts … You cheered me up a lot and your hugs are just what I like. You have a special daddy to bring you to see me. It was hard to wait to see my Katy Koala, but she was worth it! When we go hiking it will be fun, won't it? I'll try to keep up with all of you. I'll see you Friday. Love, Jo"

"Dear Melissia, It sure was fun to have pizza with you. I especially loved your sweet notes and sunshiny thoughts. Did you know God created rainbows to remind us how much he loves us and will never fail us? … You give such good hugs I'm sure to get lots better. Katy Koala seems happy with me. Your daddy is really fun, isn't he, to know a grown-up lady needs a teddy bear? See you Friday night. Love, Jo"

Ray calls to say he appreciates his card and the girls loved theirs, especially the koala stickers. He asks about my hand pain with compassion and concern. After Mom takes me to my ob-gyn and I discover I need a hysterectomy, I'm touched by her loving support as I cry. She and Rhonda both think I should've had it last week and not "messed around." I had hope. Now it's squashed.

Back in my own apartment Jessica comes over to cry about her boyfriend break-up and my up-coming hysterectomy, when Ray calls and I answer in tears. "Jessica and I are crying together. You can come join us if you like."

Ray says, "I haven't had a good cry in a long time," and we laugh. After he invites me to dinner he adds, "I'll get us two tickets to see Judy Collins, too," and I smile dreamily. "Ruth says she wants to have a picnic before the concert." *He isn't wasting any time, is he?*

At the restaurant we chat with Ray's friends, then he says, "I really like your hair." I smile, hoping he likes it when I get it re-permed. It's so easy for me curly and semi-long.

Melissia hugs me, saying, "I love you." I hug her back. "I love you, too."

Lindsey hands me a box with "love you" and a red heart in it. She, too, hugs me.

Then she declares, "We're taking Jo home with us!"

I grin, turn red, and exclaim, "Oh, you are? Okay."

Ray whispers in my ear, "When I told Lindsey I'd invited you to dinner she said, 'Oh, I'm *so* glad. I've thought about her all day and I cried for her!' It amazes me."

I tilt my head and say, my chin trembling, "They're so darling."

"I'm grateful and blessed. God gives children as the greatest blessing."

I nod and look away in pain so severe I feel like doubling over. Steroids do not bring tears to my eyes, the lack of *blessing* does. God *closed* my womb. *Perhaps I would've been a terrible mother.*

As I back away from our hug at my apartment, I think I see in his eyes the same drawing I feel—to kiss, but we don't. I journal—"Oh, the girls are precious, Lord. It would be an awesome responsibility to love and care for those two, but how can they not be hurt if Ray and I don't continue?"

The following evening Ray calls and suddenly says, "I'm dealing with some thoughts I'm not sure of right now, but I'll work them out. MS is well, frightening, because it's an unknown but—"

I interrupt, "I understand. Anyone I date needs to evaluate how much of an issue it is. I risk all the time knowing men can't handle the unpredictability."

Ray goes on, "I feel we're good friends and we might get closer, but I don't want you to think MS is what would prevent that. If we don't develop a relationship it's because we aren't compatible."

"It's only with time I'll know that's true. I ask myself why I even try. Why would I *want* anyone to put up with MS? Then I say because I'm a valuable person with a lot to give, and what's inside me is what matters. I feel blessed because MS keeps me relying on God."

"I really like you and want to get to know you and that's scary for both of us. I can back out easily because I've been hurt a lot." Ray pauses. "You see, I was married another time and have another daughter."

"Oh," is all I can say.

Ray answers my unspoken questions, "I was seventeen when I enlisted in the Marines. My girlfriend and I got pregnant, so I married her. While I was in Vietnam she wrote me a Dear John letter and divorced me. It hurt. She moved and I didn't see my daughter, Mandy, as often as I'd have liked, though I supported her through high school. She's nineteen, with a life of her own in California."

My heart aches for Ray—*two* wives rejected him.

"I've been hurt, too, Ray. But I'll never know unless I try, and I don't want a solitary life. I've been dating someone else for a while, and since I've been seeing you I've been evaluating this other guy."

Ray says, "I'm glad."

We talk about wanting time alone together since, as Ray says, laughing, "The girls *monopolize* you."

Then we say, "Good night" softly.

Chapter 11

Growing Closer, Learning More

As Ray and I sit talking with Ken and Ruth in the kitchen overlooking their property landscaped with ponderosa pines and aspen trees interspersed with huge granite boulders, I ask Ken if we can make a hot compress for my hand.

Ray asks, "Does it hurt?" I say, "Well—" Ray demands, "Yes, or *no?*"

I exclaim, "Wow, he won't let me get away with *anything*. Yes!" as Ruth howls.

Later, I explain, "I just didn't want to make a scene."

Ray cries, "You should be able to be honest with us!"

I react, "With my mother's pounding into me not to cry or gripe, be positive—I'm just trying to find a balance."

Not thirty minutes later I say, "Let's swing!"

The Peters' oldest teases me, so I respond, "I ski, why not swing?"

David's the one who commented when I hiked with Ruth and her children how well I got around. I responded, "It's because of my helps, my walking aids," so David dubbed them, "cool-aids!" and the name stuck.

I soar as high as I can, my left arm wrapped around the chain hanging onto the seat. I want to feel free and *me,* silly and carefree and young-at-heart. Ray grins as he shoots hoops nearby.

When he brings me home, after his hug and good-bye sends tingles through me, I write:

Oh God, lead me. I fear loving him and the girls and then being hurt badly, besides the girls being hurt, too. But I cannot live in fear. Ray's so assertive I think he'd overpower me, but that would be good, wouldn't it? Ruth teased that I could learn assertiveness from Ray, saying, "Jo will say yes to *anything,* especially a good time!" She's right—we've booked up next Friday through Sunday!

At the breakfast my left hand bears an odd-looking splint with my first finger's first joint held up in order to protect the tendon now freed from scar tissue. OTs will begin helping me stretch it down soon. Having heard about the upcoming hysterectomy, Elaine asks, as Ray looks on, if I've read *On Death and Dying.*[14]

I respond, "An overview was taught in our MS peer-counseling training, because though it is obviously different from accepting that you're dying, in order to live successfully one needs to grieve the losses disabilities bring and learn to adapt."

Ray remarks, "Oh, really."

Elaine, her face oozing compassion, says, "You're incredible, Jo. I know that's hard for you to hear, but it's true. I'd fold if I were you."

"To be honest," I say, snickering, "I'm about to! The steroids seem to be buzzing me worse than *ever.* I guess they're magnified by my hand discomfort."

Elaine says, "You never complain. You've always got cheer and sunshine."

Jessica adds, "*I* can't even tell you're wound up."

Ray comments, "I don't know you well enough yet to tell."

I laugh, "I'm the bottle you open and effervescence, like bubbles, escape!" *I don't have to feel guilty for saying that! You've made me like this!*

TU for taking hold of me—"I press on to take hold of that for which

Christ Jesus took hold of me … I press on toward the goal to win the prize for which God has called me heavenward in Christ Jesus" (Philippians 3:12–14). You took hold of me for a purpose—to be "transformed into *your* likeness with ever-increasing glory …" (2 Corinthians 3:18). I want to draw people to you most of all. Only glorifying you can satisfy me. I must be in you, the vine (John 15). I'm not so scared about Ray. I *can* risk. I *must* risk. I *will* risk.

I don't want to hurt Brad, but I sense God saying, "Let go." He's one of two men I've dated who asked if I prayed daily to be healed, or if I "gave up on healing." When he calls I tell him I don't feel I should be dating him any more and how sorry I am. I never wanted to hurt him.

In the morning a television interviewer requests my presence on his program in July! I'm awed by God opening this door, but a few hours later Brad calls. He's angry. "I'm just as vulnerable to be hurt as you. Don't use MS as a crutch."

Randy said the same thing.

When Ray calls I tell him about Brad's words. "Do you think your fears about rejection because of MS have a lot to do with Ron?"

I answer, "Some, though Ron had other issues, as well. Another guy I dated, for eight months, said the exact same words."

"I see. At least you're giving guys a chance." I hear tears choking Ray's voice as he says, "You *do* have so much more at stake. I feel such compassion because it seems life just hasn't been fair, and you still have the vulnerability."

"Thank you," while I'm thinking *Wow!* "I'm not asking to be handled with kid gloves but with honesty because of MS."

As Ray asks how I'm feeling, if the steroids are halting the attack, and what constitutes one, I answer all his questions, including, "An MS 'attack,' 'relapse,' or 'exacerbation' is a sudden worsening of symptoms I've had before, or the development of new neurological ones, which lasts at least twenty-four hours. Most last longer and vary in severity, and they can leave disability, or no disease progression." I admit I feel vulnerable.

Ray says, "I don't know how you handle it so well."

"It's only because of God. I *have* to trust him more, even though I'd be glad *not* to have MS."

"I admit it was a concern before I took you out. After we set it up, I met my friend Don for lunch. To be honest, because he realized he didn't know me on an emotional level, he advised me *not* to date you. He said, 'MS usually devastates the spouse.'"

I sigh sadly, "That must've been discouraging."

"It was. I told myself—just this one date. But I *still* wanted to get to know you. Even more now. Don went on to tell me his wife, Joyce, is such a blessing and a joy—"

I interrupt, "That makes me cry."

Ray continues, "Don thinks she's wonderful."

"Obviously, your friend is incredible. I've avoided saying this for fear of putting guys down, but my friends say, if there *is* someone—and I'm willing for whatever God wants—that person will be *very special.* Like you've said, 'God will have grown him to be able to handle MS and support me.'"

Ray says, "I think you feel you need to prove to me that you can do things. I *know* you can, and that's not important anyway."

Amazed at Ray's perception, I say, "I *have* felt that way. Thanks for bringing it up. That *is* a problem for me when I'm getting to know someone. Part of it's educating people that I'm not an invalid."

"I feel a little bit ashamed, but when we're out together I notice people staring and feel pity for them. Then I feel a little embarrassed. I don't want to hurt you."

"I'm glad you're honest. How do you think *I* feel? *So* conspicuous, like everyone is watching! And I know their thoughts—*What's wrong with her? I wonder if I could get what she's got. Poor thing ...* So I try to make them comfortable by smiling, holding my head high. I have nothing to be ashamed of!"

"That's the right word, Jo, 'conspicuous,' and I'm not used to that. I'll deal with it."

I tell Ray he'll have to determine how difficult it is, adding, "You're already sensitive, or you wouldn't have asked me out. And to think you learned sign language so you could hire deaf employees! That's great!" (Ray had earlier told me about having been interviewed on a TV newscast about it, and the award his company gave him.)

"Ray, I have a strong personality, strong faith. My ministry intimidates people. The MS. Problem is, others don't want to see me as needy, and I *am* sometimes. I want to be able to be weak—to *need* emotional and spiritual encouragement. Some days are so difficult. I'm exhausted easily. I say, 'This is too much, Lord. I need someone right now. If it's not to be flesh and blood, I need your extra special touch.'"

Ray says tenderly, "I know you need encouragement, Jo, and you're lonely at times. And I know you're faithful and that doesn't scare me. I'll be real with you so there are no surprises. One of the things I so appreciate about you is how real *you* are."

After our sweet good night I pray, "Lord, what a great guy. Guide totally."

When Ray and the girls come for dinner on Friday, we admit we've looked forward to it all week. I love the distinctive silk floral arrangement Ray brought for my table. We cook together, Ray putting his arm around me at times. After dinner I alternately apply ice and heat to my hand, sitting next to Ray as I exhort the girls while they learn a new game on the coffee table. Ray's tender, affectionate touches in front of them seem so natural.

When I share my concern about being a burden to my folks with my car loan he says, "I can't see you *ever* being a burden to anyone, Jo, only a blessing."

The following afternoon Ray picks me up for a barbeque. Then after a wonderful opportunity to share my testimony and sing in a morning church service, with an LPN saying she doesn't know how I have the strength to sing as I do with MS, I lie down since Ray will pick me up soon. I pray, "Father, I'm so amazed that you use *me*."

Ray drives me south, then we lounge on a blanket with Ken and Ruth near the outdoor stage talking, touching shoulders, hinting at being affectionate. (Ruth tells me the next day Ken just wanted to tell Ray, "Kiss her!") I'm immersed as a long-time fan of Judy Collins, but realize *I'm glad she can do this, but I'm glad I get to do it with you, Jesus.* Afterwards, Ray asks when *he* can see me in concert, so I give him a date in a couple weeks.

When he brings me home I offer him apples, cheese and crackers while I get some relief from the painful swelling, icing my wrist and hand. Then I curl up on the couch with my legs under me as I look at Ray turned towards me. I ask about his background and he teases me about being nosey.

But I protest, "I want to know you!"

Ray takes a breath, then unfolds a story I don't expect. His parents were both alcoholics, so uninvolved in their six children's lives that the kids were put in foster homes twice, once for almost two years. The five brothers and one sister weren't even in the same home. I gasp. As the oldest, Ray was responsible for his siblings, and if his dad was displeased, he smacked Ray. Sometimes he hit Ray for no reason at all. My heart contracts with sadness.

I look into his soulful eyes as he continues, "I had no real encouragement, affirmation or love. I've come a *long* way to not let that cause me problems. I have to parent myself to maintain good ethics because I didn't have good role models. When my mom remarried after my dad died of cirrhosis of the liver, her new alcoholic husband had some money, so I got a new car. I thought that would make people like me."

He shakes his head and goes on, "After being in Vietnam with the Marines I lived like a hippie for a few years. I got my GED and an associate degree in college after that. I want to go back and get my bachelor's."

I shake my head compassionately. "I'm blessed to have you in my life, Ray."

He reaches across the back of the couch to touch my arm, "I went to the breakfast to meet women. I want to feel useful in a relationship."

I look at Ray with wide eyes and nod.

"I really like you, Jo. You're a quality person—about the most quality woman I know! When I saw you I wanted to take you out. You were mesmerizing in that black hat with the netting. I think it's *amazing* that I feel so comfortable so quickly with you. I wouldn't have told people those things six years ago and very few people now."

"I'm proud of what you've done and I think you should be."

Ray thanks me and I say, "You could've chosen to be just like your parents, and yet you've shown your children both love and discipline."

Ray says, "I know I need to present God to them."

How beautiful, Lord.

He goes on, "You know, that's why I became a Christian. A friend from work invited me to a James Dobson film series about the family at his church. I realized I couldn't be a good father without God. I became a Christian following a film and began going to church without my wife."

Tears fill my eyes.

"But I blow it and get mad at the girls sometimes."

"Do you ask their forgiveness? That shows them good role modeling, too."

Ray nods and I decide to ask, "How did you feel walking around that crowd with me? Conspicuous?"

Ray answers, "Not as much, but it doesn't come naturally, Jo. It doesn't matter that you aren't healthy, I see *you*. And you have incredible integrity. I respect that *so much*. People trade it easily. What you really have Jo, is *who you are*. Nobody can take that away from you."

My mouth is half-open, "Where did you learn that, about integrity?"

Ray answers, "From the Lord a couple years ago."

We talk about growing in wisdom and I say, "It's important to me that a guy *want* to grow as a Christian, and accepts MS may be God's plan for me. I know you pray for me to be healed—"

Ray cuts in, "It may not be God's will, Jo. I know that."

"I'm glad. If he can't accept it, someone would get really tired of hearing my story of how God is sufficient in the midst of living with it." Ray agrees.

We talk a little more then he says, "Well, I'll go now, okay?"

"I guess it's time."

He puts his arm around me and lightly touches his lips to mine so I move into his arms for a hug. When he gets up I ask how tall he is. "Six-foot-three."

We move to the door and I reach my arms around him, his encircle me, and I bend my head back to give *him* a light kiss. After I close the door, I lean against it and sigh with a far-away look in my eyes and a smile spreading across my face.

Lord, I'm really attracted to this man. He's come so far. He loves you. Wants your will though he admits the world is tempting. He knows his weaknesses. He has goals and dreams, and feels capable of reaching them. When he compliments me I *want* to believe him. *He really likes me.* I want to hug him, he's so wonderful, (and good-looking!) He admits he analyzes possible scenarios, then realizes you're in control. I do the same. I'm a little afraid, but not as much. How wonderful it would be to share joy and sorrow with him. To believe in each other. I've always been surprised guys asked me out, Lord. Don't let me jump ahead in my thoughts. I want to have the integrity Ray sees in me, to be like Paul who writes in 2 Corinthians 1:12 that he conducted himself in the world and with you in a holy and sincere way according to your grace.

I come home from shopping the next afternoon to a message, "Hello beautiful! Give me a call at work."

I shudder with delight as I dial his number. He tells me he's checked into tandems at a bike shop. *He's thinking of what we can do together!* Ray tells me to be careful as I drive to the airport to pick up Swedish friends and says, "G'bye," with caring.

Once I pick up Oddvar and Rita and their daughters, we meet the Peters family, Ray, Lindsey, and Melissia for a picnic.

As we all begin a hike Lindsey says, "Jo, you can't do this part!"

I retort teasingly, "Oh? Just watch me! Don't say, 'I can't'" as I make it up the narrow path.

Later, I pray, "Lord, is it pride? Is it wrong to resent others suggesting I can't do something? Do I bother them with my 'Never give up' and 'I'll try anything' attitude? Especially when I *know* there are things I can't do—like breaking the scar tissue that's already building up in my hand and wrist? Help my hand not to be like it was before the surgery."

When I tell Ruth about driving my friends over Trail Ridge Road as I cried out to God for strength in my fatigue, I find out she and Ray talked a long time. Ruth says he's not bothered by others' stares, he just wants to be with me. He wants to see more, not less, of me, as it happens sometimes when you're around someone.

"Ruth, it's mutual," I interject.

Ray said I came into his life when he was lonely and looking, and he's amazed at how great and comfortable it is. Ruth told him she can't help seeing anyone I date as a prospective husband, and he told her he can't help thinking that either, when it's someone he cares about. When she said my mom was concerned the girls would be too much for me, he said he was, too. Then mom met and fell in love with all three of them and she has no concerns. Ray told her, "That's good."

Ruth asked if he'd like to go to dinner with them for my birthday, and he said he'd already cancelled a rafting trip to take me out, though he hadn't told me yet. *Wow, he cancelled fun plans for* me!

When Ray calls from work to discuss making plans without the Malneses, he says, "I may hurt you sometimes because of the way I feel about something, but two people don't always have to agree."

"I know. I haven't been offended yet."

He continues, "I'm not a people pleaser anymore. If you stay around, I just want you to know that."

Surprised, I respond, "I'm not going anywhere."

Ray says gently, "I spent seven years trying to make over my wife, and she did me—it doesn't work."

"I agree. I just want to be me and let you be you. I *do* want to learn about my attitude or the way I do things that might not be right, and that may need to come from another person."

Ray sounds exposed as he says, "I want to be open, but the hardest thing for me is to admit there's a better way. It's *really* hard."

I respond gently, "God uses it to hone us, to make us more Christ-like."

He says, "I guess so."

The Malneses and I are at my folks' when in walks Melissia practically hidden by two dozen red, pink, salmon, and white roses! *He had the courage and determination to give these to me in front of my family!* Melissia and Lindsey dote on me, hugging and kissing me frequently.

Ray notices my dad sitting alone and whispers to me, "We should talk to him." Then we notice Grandmother alone and chat with her.

I'm so impressed by Ray's sensitivity that I list in his Father's Day card all the attributes I see in him, adding:

> "The roses are opening up beautifully, just as I like to see my life and the lives of others open up when we risk by giving of ourselves to others—something I say before I sing 'The Rose.' I thoroughly enjoy the way you treat me! Even warning each other of our flaws we've yet to see for fear we'll frighten each other off—it all seems so natural ... God bless you more than you ask or imagine (Ephesians 3:20). Love, Jo"

The following evening at Ray's home, Lindsey and Melissia point out their mother's house across the street. Ray had told me he moved into her neighborhood when she left because he wanted them near their mother. Since he cried for his mom at night in foster homes, he wanted his daughters to be close to their mom. Now Lindsey and Melissia can go over whenever they want, and she does have certain times, like tonight, to have them. They want to stay with us, but Ray encourages them to go to their mom's when he notices the movie is two hours long. We lie back on the over-sized couch and put our feet up on the maple coffee table and munch popcorn. After awhile Ray turns to kiss me. *Oh, it is so tender, yet passionate.*

I soon say, "We need to cool down," and he agrees. We roll the movie back.

Ray says, "It's so comfortable being with you it's almost scary. You're really beautiful, you know. You were so cute when I called to ask you out and you said, 'Well, that's a possibility.'"

He laughs and I smile. I lie down on the couch and lay my legs over his lap.

"You have a lot to be grateful for, Ray, two wonderful daughters who love you so much. You'll have a great Father's Day. I wanted children so badly I cried at friends' baby showers, now I need a hysterectomy in August."

Ray squeezes and strokes my arm.

"It's a little hard. I feel I really missed out, but I'll accept it."

Ray responds gently, "God has something else for you, Jo."

When Ray kisses me at my door later I sense he's shared my pain in the same way I've shared his.

I receive the health insurance stub back, which I sent to Ron for payment, with a note telling me his folks are visiting. He writes that he hopes my surgery will resolve the particular needs I face. Ray's attitude of forgiveness prompted me to pray about being a blessing to Ron this time. I had written—"Ron, I thank God and you for your consistent financial help. Hope this finds you with God's precious love wrapped around you. Jo." After reading his note I journal:

> As I read in 2 Corinthians 2:10—"And what I have forgiven … I have forgiven in the sight of Christ for your sake, in order that Satan might not outwit us. For we are not unaware of his schemes." I'm glad I haven't given Satan an opportunity, just as Ray hasn't given Satan one either by forgiving his former wife.

After the girls swim and I help them dry off and prepare to shower in my cozy bathroom Ray says, "I'm amazed at how easily and quickly the girls have taken to you!"

"It's wonderful. I didn't know what to expect, but I just *love* them."

Ray smiles as he leans on my kitchen counter, "I thank God for putting you in my life, Jo. I'm so grateful. Not just any woman—you! I miss you. I can hardly wait to see you, but when I'm close I feel slightly uneasy. I can't tell you why, but it's inside me. It's not anything *you're* doing. That's why I can't express my feelings sometimes."

"It seems you're expressing them *pretty well*." I pause. "Is it MS?"

Ray answers quickly, "No, I really don't think so. God's helped me deal with that. I feel it's taken care of. I see you, Jo, who you are *inside*."

"I had to ask."

Ray nods and I cautiously proceed, "I suspect—I think—I'm not *tell-ing* you I know this, but maybe you feel *too* comfortable with me and that makes you a little nervous."

Ray nods again, "It could be. You make me feel so *special*. I'm not used to that!"

"And you make *me* feel special. Well, I guess there's only one cure, that's to not see me. The alternative is to work it out."

Ray says, "I don't run away. I deal with things," and I smile.

After dinner, which is full of fun chatter from Lindsey and Melissia, Ray puts his arms around me from behind in a hug as he asks, "Is it okay if I give Jo a hug in front of you?"

I add, "We hug you a lot, too."

They say in unison, "Sure."

Ray begins helping and I say, "You have to realize I've lived alone for almost three years. I take my trash out on a luggage carrier or in my car to the dumpster!"

He shakes his head, "I can't understand how you've done it!"

I shrug and respond, "When I told Judie Amen about you today she said something profound. She suggested maybe we get along so well because we're both survivors. We won't give up. I admire that in you."

Before leaving Ray invites me to join him and the girls in their Friday night ritual. He gives me a hug and quick kiss in front of the girls. As we say good-bye each of the girls hug me and say, "I love you," with my return-ing the same.

Lindsey runs back from the car to thank me and from the car she yells, "I love you!"

Ray calls when he arrives home, inviting me to Hal and Peg's for a barbecue with his old "assertiveness training" group. As we talk about feel-ings again I say, "I think what you're feeling are fears of risking because of feeling comfortable and caring."

Ray says softly, "You're probably right. The fear of being vulnerable."

"I have the same fears, but you and your children are such blessings,

I won't give up the opportunities to be with you until they're no longer offered. Even though I know I'm God's special, unrepeated miracle of creation, I *still can't understand why I'm so blessed to have you three in my life.* I know I have some self-esteem problems."

Tenderness fills Ray's voice. "That's okay. It just makes you more human and real."

"I'm trying to just enjoy and risk."

"That's good. In the car Lindsey said, 'You know, Dad, I think I like Jo better than any of your other girlfriends.' I said, 'You know, Lindsey, I think I do, too.' Jo, I really do like you *a lot.* Have a good night's sleep. I look forward to talking and being with you soon."

I lie on my stomach on my rose comforter. "Lord, I think we both love each other and are afraid to say it. We want to be vulnerable, but can't. We want to risk. We enjoy each other so much. Lead us."

Chapter 12

Love Breeds Fear

When I pick up the phone Ray says, "I was thinking so much about you I just decided to call! What about going to Ouray?"

I ask, "When are the girls free?"

He answers, "Can you go in late July?"

I protest, "But the girls will be with their mom in California on vacation."

"I just want *us* to go," Rays says, as I *see* his smiling eyes.

My mouth drops open. Finally, I say, "Sounds great, but what about sleeping arrangements?"

"I'll pay for separate rooms." I protest his paying, but he says we'll talk more, leaving both of us excited.

In the morning Jessica tells me she's getting baptized.

I can personalize these verses in Jessica's card—"You yourself are my letter written on my heart, known and read by everybody. You show that you are a letter from Christ, the results of my ministry not written with ink but with the Spirit of the living God, not on tablets of stone but on tablets of human hearts" (2 Corinthians 3:2–3). I'm so privileged to share your love with others, Lord!

On Friday night we feast on Mexican food, then head into the mall. In a candy store Ray buys bubble gum jellybeans, saying, "They're my favorite."

Lindsey and Melissia giggle, hold my hand, skip away, and return for a hug. Back at Ray's Melissia brings me ice water while Ray puts on our favorite jazz guitar music. I lean back into Ray's arms and gaze out the window at my beloved mountains, saying, "This is wonderful."

Later I write—"Lord, is he uneasy and afraid? I am. Loving without risking is impossible. *Grow my faith in your plan for me as I risk with Ray.*"

Two days later on my birthday I journal:

Psalm 139 is for me. You knew me *before* I was born, God. You love me so much I cry tears of joy. You knew what my life would be like before I lived it. That I'd become hurt, wounded, and ill, but you would be all I need. TU you for keeping me from killing myself three years ago so I can enjoy another day of life with you.

Then I sing for my first wedding since Anne and Dave's. *Oh Lord, TU for your joy and peace. I didn't feel hurt or cynical or bitter.* After taking a short rest I begin dressing for my date.

When Ray knocks on my door bearing red roses and a card he says, "You're not your bubbly self. Are you okay?"

I read the touching sentiment in the card and lean into his arms for a hug and kiss.

Ray says, "You sure look beautiful." I smile and say, "Thanks. I was really nervous because you've never seen me dressed up before." He laughs. "I *knew* something was up. Well, you shouldn't have worried!"

During our dinner with Ken and Ruth—who are as giddy as me—I *must* be glowing. Back at my apartment, Ray says, "I ask myself, 'What does she see in you?' but I just consider myself blessed."

I squeeze his hand, saying, "Reread those cards."

Ray's smile tugs at my heart, "I don't consider our relationship casual anymore. I'm not just thinking about wanting to see you, but what that really means."

He pauses and looks deep into my eyes.

My heart hammers as he asks, "Do you know what I want to say right now?"

I stutter, "I-I think so."

Ray urges, "What?"

"Huh-uh. You tell me."

"I think I love you, Jo."

I kiss Ray lightly. "I think I love you, too."

Neither of us can contain our smiles as I ask, "How long have you wanted to say that?"

"About a week. I don't think—I *know* I love you, Jo."

"I've wanted to tell you for about that long." I stifle a laugh as I say, "Actually, this is embarrassing, I wrote the night of our first date—'Wow! I'm smitten!'"

Ray bursts out laughing.

My voice is almost a whisper. "I realized I loved you when I was just looking at you."

He says, "I realized when you weren't even around."

We both agree we've become emotionally attached quickly, yet we grin when we agree that Peg will be happy!

After my concert the following evening, old friends introduce themselves warmly to Ray. He hugs me with tears as he says, "It was the best concert I've ever attended because I was ministered to."

He murmurs, "I still feel the same as last night."

I say softly, "So do I."

Ray continues, "I feel God's answering my prayer to get closer to him and you're being used for that growth."

Tears fill my eyes. "I'm so glad."

When Ray calls later I'm ready for bed. I say, "I'm glad you accept my ministry of vulnerability. Some of my family members say, 'The past is past, go on.'"

"But you're being *real,* and people relate to that and grow! It's *great.* I see God using you, Jo. It feels like he's evaluating me, saying, 'I've given her this ministry, Ray. Are you in the way?' I love you and enjoy being with you, then I think *Jo may not be able to do these things through the years,* and tell myself it doesn't really matter because the Jo I love is inside. I feel you would communicate things out if the MS got worse."

I nod as if Ray can see me, saying, "Yes, and I'm the type of person who *never* gives up. I'm not trying to sell myself, but when I couldn't walk, I *still* wanted to ride horseback with a friend! I've always wanted to get the most out of life and always will."

Ray says, "I do have to consider the girls—will their needs be met?"

I respond, "I understand."

Ray goes on, "I analyze things, and as they come up I'm working them through. I haven't realized any big hurdles yet."

"If you do, you'll tell me?"

"Yes, you'll know. I'll never go into marriage again without a lot of pre-marital counseling. I don't want things to be found out later."

"I agree."

"And when I get married this time is forever."

"I've told the Lord not to put *anyone* in my life if I'm not going to be able to make it last forever." *But both Ray and I wanted our marriages to last, Lord. We didn't give up.*

He declares, "I want a relationship with someone who will love me whether I'm *right or wrong.* I want to share life with someone, joys *and* sorrows."

"I know exactly what you mean."

Ray adds, "Paul says if you're burning with passion then you'd better marry!"

I laugh at his candor.

His voice softens, "I just think it's so great that it's mutual. On the way to your concert Lindsey said, 'I wish Jo were my mommy,' and I asked her, 'Why?' She said, 'Because I love her.' I asked, 'Why do you love her?' 'Because she's so nice and she cares about me and she loves me.'"

I tear up, "Ray, how sweet. Thanks for telling me."

Ray says, "I love you."

"I love you, too. That's scary to say."

Ray agrees, adding, "I love things about you, Jo, such that I feel the more I know you, the more I'll love you."

I melt into my comforter, unable to move, "I feel the same."

When we meet for lunch the following day I give Ray a card to read while he flies to Boston tomorrow with photos of me. After I hand him MS information about fatigue and emotional aspects he says, "Great! I've intended on asking for this."

We mouth "I love you" as he drives away, and I'm soaring in my heart. Later I journal our conversation:

> Ray admits having trouble asking forgiveness, but said he gets around to it eventually. He blurts things out. I told him, "I *don't* want to be harsh like Mom, but I have to turn off negative tapes in order to say something I know will sound profound." I told him I appreciate his strength. Ray said, "When my wife left, besides counseling, I read books by Chuck Swindoll and James Dobson on how godly men should be." I said, "That's great."

I just have to tell Inga and Ruben how things are going with Ray, so I call them at Solskinet. They're excited, yet no matter how happy I am, I deal once again with fears:

> If I need to learn through Ray's rejection, use it, Lord, to make me who you want me to be. Misbelief—I couldn't be trusted to be a good mother because I've never been one and because I have MS. Truth—I can learn. And MS could be the best thing that ever happened to them because of sensitivity to others.

Now it seems I'm suffocating under a load poured over me by a dump truck—my "new" used car needs an entire valve job! I cry out to God, "Somehow I *know* you'll provide my needs," as I *literally* cry. Then I tear open the note I just received:

> "Dear Beloved Jo, My infinite gratitude to our Lord of love for your glorious ministry. Such a great heart! Marcus, my husband, wouldn't listen to your tape, saying, "She's more wonderful than her tape! There's so much

heart in her songs." My youngest, Jeda, said, "She's so happy!" A wonderful tribute to your uplifting, indomitable spirit. As for me, I'm more into the Word since knowing you and have more courage and acceptance of my own hidden disability. Thank you, Jo for being you. Lovingly, Jasmine"

I implore, "But the warrior is a child!" tears covering my face. "So lovingly you let me be a child crying out in pain as you enfold me in your embrace. In my head I trust you with this monetary problem—I need it to be heart-knowledge. TU for this note and TU for loving me."

The following day I drive to the mall to purchase bubble gum jellybeans, placing the bag in a coffee mug pictured with a cute, overwhelmed bear next to a pile of paperwork that says, "Bear with me." After wrapping it in bear-y cellophane I write in the card—"Dear Ray, Welcome back!" In a letter I list affirmations of Ray's character, and a list of how he's meeting my needs. Then I pray, "Lord, show me if I should really give this to Ray, I don't want to scare him or get ahead of your will!" In the morning I put the letter in the card. I drive many miles to Ray's office. I timidly ask the receptionist to place it on Ray's desk.

She says, "He's going to love this!" and I sigh with relief.

After my dinner of nachos, I answer the phone to hear Ray say, "Hi, beautiful!"

Surprised, I ask, "Where are you?"

"New York. I have one hour before my flight leaves, and I missed you so much I had to call!" I sigh. He continues, "I wish my flight got in earlier. You're on my way home."

"When do you arrive?"

"Midnight." Beyond all reason I say, "Well … I guess—"

Reading my mind, Ray says, "You should get your sleep."

"I can rest tomorrow. I'd love to see you."

"I'd *love* to see *you*," he says excitedly.

I lie on the couch listening for his car and meet him at the door. He swallows me in a hug, then plops next to me on the couch, saying, "I *really* needed to see you."

"I love being this unconventional."

Ray says, "I thought about you all the time."

"Yesterday, I talked about you all day."

Ray leans close to my face, saying, "I love you, Jo," and kisses me thoroughly.

I lie down on the couch with my legs over his lap as he says, "I enjoyed reading the material." I say, "Enjoyed?"

Ray nods, "Sure. Didn't you think I'd read it?"

"Yes—"

"Thought it would scare me?" He shakes his head. "Not at all. MS isn't the worst thing you could have. I don't think it makes you any less of a woman. Give me more to read every so often."

Ray begins the following day with a message, "You're so thoughtful. Thanks for the mug and candy." Since he doesn't say anything about my letter I wonder all day if I went too far. When I bring it up later he says, "It *was* vulnerable. I appreciate the affirmation. I'll try to live up to it."

As I explain my car financial struggles and how I want to trust God Ray says, "I really admire you because you're so trusting."

I smirk, "It isn't always easy. I asked the Lord, 'Why do I get to trust you for finances and health, etc. daily? I want to be more like Jesus than anything, so keep me having to trust you.'"

Ray smiles, saying, "You have such character and integrity which I admire. It gives you self-esteem, self-image."

As if a plane flies by with a banner, I suddenly realize Ray's correct and say, "You're right! When Ron tore me down I prayed to be Christ-like, and he re-built me! I felt I'd done all I could before the divorce. I guess I never looked at character and integrity as something I asked for, but God's producing that in me. It's interesting, Judie Amen said, 'I know you're seeking God in this, Jo, because of your integrity.'"

Ray says, "You show people in concerts how to live with integrity."

Later, I read 2 Corinthians 5:17 and write—"If any man is in Christ he is a new creation; the old has gone, the new come!' I can be a person of character and integrity because I'm a new creation in you! TU Jesus! I'm your ambassador with a message of reconciliation—what purpose you give me."

When Ray picks me up to meet his friends from the former group at Hal and Peg's he says, "I never get to listen to your album—the girls play it constantly. I think God has his hand in this."

He looks over at me as I say, "I agree."

Ray's attentive at the barbeque, wanting me to feel comfortable. Later he says he went to singles' for a purpose—to meet women, which is now fulfilled, and I respond, "And women are mad at *me.*"

He laughs. As we continue talking, I wonder what's going on.

In the morning I ask to come by and talk with him tonight. I hug the girls, then Ray and I sit on the couch. I say, "I wanted to put my arm around you last night when you said you'd been hurt in every relationship. I wanted to tell you I don't want to hurt you, but to love and share life with you. I was scared because I'm risking so much, caring about all of you."

Ray sighs, "You can't do anything about this, Jo. It's my problem. I've had a lot of rejection from my childhood on. It causes me to be scared and draw back."

I touch Ray's arm compassionately, saying, "Your assertiveness intimidates me so I sometimes respond with defensiveness, but I'm learning. I fear your strength, but I love it and want it and need it. I got to the breakfast today and knew I wanted to be with you, wherever you were."

Ray smiles slightly, loosening up as he caresses my arm. He says, "I haven't felt peace about our relationship lately."

"I sensed that."

"I know I like you a lot, and love you in some ways—love is an ongoing process."

I nod, saying, "Right, you grow in love."

Ray goes on, "But I've been concerned about how fast the emotional side happened. It's wonderful, but I realize I don't *know* you."

Ray's serious face causes fear to grab hold with the tight grip of a clamp, as if to cut off the blood flow of love to my heart.

He says, "I thought today about whether I want to change our relationship. See less of you or see others."

The clamp halts the flow and I feel light-headed.

Ray states, "I decided if I'm going to get to know you, I need to do things *with* you. I think the trip will be a good time to get to know each other."

I sputter, "I was going to ask if you still wanted to go."

"Yes. I'm looking at lots of things. The girls enter in, but that's not the only issue. I ask *what do I want?* The girls need someone, but do I just want help bringing them up? I want to be fair. I go slowly."

I try to breathe and say, "I do, too. I've been surprised at how quickly we've grown emotionally, and I respect you for thinking that shouldn't be emphasized. If you decide to see other women it's only fair that you *tell me*, because I'm investing a lot."

Ray says, "I don't have any grand design, but I'll tell you. It's nice to have the warm fuzzies and all, but relationships are made of good communication."

I feel a little worn-out and scared as I say, "I'm glad for the talk."

"Me, too. See, sometimes you need to be a rescuer. I don't always bring things up," his smile barely discernible.

Then Ray lists things he likes about me before he says, "There's hardly anything I don't like. You have a little bit of wanting to be in control at times, and because I want that, we'll probably butt heads and need to compromise, but I also like that in you."

I smile tightly, saying, "I can compromise too easily. I know my wanting to be in control, or appearing to want to be, comes from my improved self-esteem—I have an opinion."

"That's good. Too much compromise comes from a low self-image."

I ask him what he meant by "God being in this" and he responds, "I *do* believe God wants me in this relationship, but I want to enjoy getting to know you!"

Then we get some minor issues off our chests like my mothering him about too much sugar and fatty foods. We laugh a little, and he walks me to my car, kisses me, and I say, "I just want you to know I love you."

Ray responds, "I love you, too."

I drive home with thoughts tumbling one over another and collapse journaling:

> Does Ray need someone *so* together and unafraid of risking that she will *not* let him reject her or give messages of confusion? I *think* Ray's worth it. If I'm to lose this relationship, I'll bear it and give you glory. I count *all* things as loss except knowing you as my Lord (Philippians 3:8). I want to know you *more*. I'm at *your* mercy, not Ray's. My worth doesn't depend on whether I meet Ray's or the girls' needs. You love me. I'm your special, unique, unrepeated miracle of creation *as I am.*

In the morning I get back to ministry—vocalize, prepare for an outreach event, and an upcoming TV program. I have to be so careful not to overdo with my limited energy. I'm afraid I could become more disabled.

Tears fill my eyes when I hear Ray's sensitive tone on his message, indicating he knows I might be feeling insecure. Then Lindsey calls, saying she's tried several times.

"Leave a message. I love to hear your sweet voice."

She asks, "When are we going to have our day together without Daddy? I leave for California next Saturday!"

I say, "It's hard when you're in year-round school."

"Yeah, maybe when I get back."

Then Ray gets on the phone, "I've been sick for three days. I kinda need to apologize for how grumpy I've been and how I let it make me think there was something wrong with our relationship. I *really* appreciate you coming over last night to talk about it."

I remark, "I *had* to."

He asks more about my surgery then says, "It doesn't seem fair."

"Last year was so good I couldn't deal with all the blessings and this year whammy! I'm asking people to pray I don't have another MS attack."

Ray says, "I know you don't like steroids and the 'moon face' they give you, but you handled them well. I got to know you then and was really attracted to you. At least I know I can handle the worst times."

I'm thinking *that wasn't the worst* while Ray continues, "Jo, to be honest, I've been thinking about other girls I'm attracted to that don't have an illness. It sure would be easier. Then I think *what about hidden emotional problems?* Those would be worse. At least with MS you know the risks and decide to handle it."

I rub my left eye and cheek subconsciously, "I appreciate how you're thinking this through."

Ray cries, "I do care, but I never expected this to go anywhere. I thought I'd go out with you one time after talking to Don. Told myself, *be honest, you don't need this.*"

Feeling discouraged and defensive, I say, "I understand if it's too much."

"I don't want you to think I'm somebody special. It takes work. I was praying for someone to share spiritual things with and had no idea it would be a girlfriend!"

I respond, "I can't exist without sharing this way."

Ray says, "I feel you're in my life to cause me to grow in some way."

All my insecurities rise up within me. "Maybe I'm in your life to help you see how to experience joy in the midst of anything. That's what others tell me they learn."

Inwardly I sigh. "I believe this is hard for men, but no one can permanently be in my life who doesn't see God has given him the privilege along with the burden. Otherwise he may become angry with God and me. I want a relationship where someone will share MS—it's ours, *not* mine."

Ray says he needs to get things done.

It hurts to know loving me takes so much effort. Do I have to be afraid of another rejection notice? If so, let it happen *now.* I don't want it to hurt worse than it already would for any of us. I feel like giving up. I need Ray to show sensitivity tomorrow night.

When I pick up Lindsey and Melissia from their mom's they run to the car. As we drive home Lindsey looks at me compassionately, asking, "How could your husband leave you just because you have MS?"

I smile slightly and say, "It wasn't just MS."

Her face perks up as she states, "My dad doesn't want to leave you because you have MS!" My heart squeezes because I know more than she does.

Lindsey blurts out, "What names would your children have if you had them?"

I answer, "Well, I only thought about a girl's name, but she would've been called Joy because that's what she would bring me."

Lindsey tilts her head thoughtfully, saying, "Soooo, you wanted a girl, huh?"

When Ray arrives we hug as he says, "I was looking forward to this."

I put my head on his chest and agree with him.

He asks the girls if they're going to be at their mom's on July 4 after our hike, teasing, "It's okay with me if you let me be alone with Jo."

Lindsey teases back, "You *always* want to be alone with Jo."

Ray asks, "Does that bother you?"

Lindsey says, "No, I just want to be alone with her, too."

Melissia says with a frown, "It bothers *me*." When we ask her why, she says she doesn't know, can't say, then abruptly retorts, "You don't love us!"

Ray and I both state, "That's not true. We *do* love you."

Lord, give her peace.

On the 4th over breakfast, I see Melissia fighting jealousy even though I know she loves me. All three of them help me along the trail as I exclaim about God's amazing creation. Later, while eating dinner at Ray's, Melissia fights to sit next to me.

As I lie down on the couch, overheated from the hike and Ray's warm house, he sets a box fan to blow on me and brings ice water. He tells about a friend whose sister had done fine with MS till four years ago and is now in a care facility at age forty-nine.

I ask, "How does that make you feel?"

Ray says, "Scared," and he looks it. Ray continues sadly, "It's the unknown that's so frightening. I want more information. I don't know enough. I wish it weren't such an issue for others, or me, but it is." He pats and rubs my leg.

I sense a familiar black hole of despair threatening to suck me in. I feel like saying *I knew when you said it wouldn't matter you hadn't thought it through.*

Ray interrupts my silence, crying out, "I'm not afraid of *your* attitude with your dependence on the Lord. I'm afraid I might *hurt you* by not being able to handle the MS." His voice lowers, tears glistening his eyes, "I can't promise you I *can* handle it, but I promise I'll try."

I shrug, "Thanks. I feel so frustrated. Like giving up. It's my cross to bear and it's painful. Sometimes I'm ashamed because I have a pity-party."

Ray says tenderly, "I've come a ways. It doesn't bother me at all to be with you now."

Inside I sigh, *Gee, Lord, wonderful.*

We lounge on his deck, fireworks displays flashing brilliant colors in numerous places. The girls come and go, giving hugs and kisses before they romp away to hold sparklers at their mom's.

Ray says, "I'm going to pay for the rooms on our trip," and I argue but he urges, "I *want* to."

What a sweetheart. Our friends seem to trust and want us to have time alone. We know we want to be pure before God, but admit we're really attracted to each other.

As we talk about the girls Ray reveals, "I can be impatient, like a drill sergeant, but I had no discipline and wasted a lot of life because of it." I ponder how Ray's shortness with them bothered me, but I think I softened it a bit. *It's so hard for one parent all the time,* I reason.

Even with stressful talk about MS I journal a list of TUs at home and pray:

> Lord, I know in my weakness you're strong. Can Ray look at sharing responsibility, pain and suffering, as an opportunity for you to be made strong in his weakness? That's the only way a man will have peace with MS and live with joy, not terror. Show him. If it's your will for me to be used in Ray's life just to bring him closer to you and to bless him and

the girls, but there won't be deeper commitment, I *will* praise you. I give myself for Ray's growth, a sacrifice of praise (Hebrews 13:15).

Ray and I spend an absolutely divine day full of caring, teasing and laughter, then I don't hear from him for days. I sense him pulling back, and my journal fills with concerns about whether this is too stressful. Finally, I call Peg. She suggests I need to hold him accountable by sharing my feelings, because I shouldn't remain in turmoil. So, I take a huge breath, say a prayer, "Prepare Ray's heart to be open and receptive," and dial his number.

I explain how different our relationship feels, like he's pulled back, just as he said he could. "It triggers my fear of rejection. It would be better if you just said, 'I need some time and space, and may not call regularly.'"

Ray states, "I don't think we have a relationship."

I'm shocked, but manage to say, "Friendship can be killed by fear, too."

Frustration fills his voice. "I need time. My biggest fear is I don't know whether *I'm* capable of having a relationship."

"Listen carefully," I say softly. "This is not blame, but a question. Could all of your past rejection and fear of abandonment cause you to pull away?"

Ray says angrily, "You're bringing up a lot of feelings!"

"I'm sorry that hurts. It's not my intention."

Ray answers with a sigh, "I have areas I need space in, and encouragement, and you don't want to be a rescuer, but I guess I need help. I love you and think I'll love you more, but I may not be able to be in a relationship."

Ray finally says, "Just talking to you tonight caused me to know how much I care about you and it brought up some pretty deep emotions. You're able to make me feel things I should be able to identify, and maybe work through. It's been hard to have these conversations, but I appreciate you calling. I know you were very vulnerable. I could have told you 'Bug off!' I think we're doing okay, Jo. You're just going to have to be patient. Ask me if something is wrong when it happens. Confront me."

Do I hear 'Don't give up on me?' I'm glad I called. Ray cares, he's just afraid.

A few days later Lindsey, Melissia and I spend the afternoon together. They both say they like me better than anyone their daddy's dated because I *want* to spend time with them, and I care about them.

I cry, "I *love* being with you! You're blessings from God in my life, and I *love you*," as I hug each of them fiercely, while they grin.

When Ray arrives at my place he puts his arms around me, his head against mine, and thanks me for calling. "Good things aren't always happy, sometimes they're hard. Have you read *Caring Enough to Confront?*"[15]

I chuckle, "I have it."

After we kiss I say, "I've got to tell you, I don't kiss friends like this."

It's his turn to chuckle, saying, "You're right. This *is* more than a casual friendship. It's just hard for me to admit."

I nod, "I know it's scary, but look at the benefits!"

I tell Ray what the girls said. He shakes his head as he says, "I wouldn't let the few other women I've dated take the girls places. I didn't want them to get attached and hurt."

I smile with a turned head, "Then I must be privileged."

"You are."

The following morning Ray takes me to his church. Ruth and Ken nod happily. After we stand through one praise song Ray suggests we sit. I love how sensitive he is to my level of strength. We spend the afternoon looking at houses since he wants to move. I ask if he'd like to take me to the TV program I'm to be on this week.

"I need prayer support. I've had lunch with the interviewer, and he seems to think if everyone isn't healed it's a faith issue."

Ray and I begin looking at verses together and eventually he says, "People need to look at healing as to whether it's *God's* will, not just what *they* want. I pray for God to use you however he wants."

Suddenly Ray's expression softens, and the growing warmth from his gaze makes my cheeks rosy as he says, "I don't know what would've happened if you hadn't called. I'm *so* glad you did. I need an assertive woman."

I look at Ray with love and hurt as tears fill his eyes and he struggles with words. "I realized how much you mean to me and thought, *Ray this is one special woman. She's worth the risk!* I love you, Jo. I want you to know I've dealt with the MS and we can just work on our relationship. I love you *just the way you are.* You're *exactly* what I want!"

"Exactly?"

"I wouldn't change a thing! And I like having you with my children."

I respond, "That's so wonderful," as my heart nearly bursts with joy.

Ray tells me he talked again to his friend whose sister is doing badly, and discovered it had to do with her attitude of giving up. Though that saddened Ray, he realizes I'll never do that. He tells me he loves my appreciation of beauty.

"Mom gave me that. We did a lot of jeeping and taking drives in the mountains. I had a good home."

"You must have. You're really mature emotionally, and it didn't come from the past few years."

Later I realize I disagree. I learned from my growing relationship with God, books, and all the counseling I've had lately.

It's hard to say goodbye this evening. We've crossed a threshold, it seems, moving us onto another level. It's also the start of many calls. He can't wait until our trip on Friday, and neither can I!

Chapter 13

Happiness, a Sad Hysterectomy, and Ray's Doubts

Ray stands at my door, beaming, plants a happy smack on my lips, and picks up my luggage. After several pit stops he teases about opening up restrooms for ladies across the country. I tease that I should invest in toilet paper companies' stock.

As we drive over Wolf Creek Pass in Southwestern Colorado on the way to Durango I "Oooo" and "Ahhh," crying, "I love God's creation!"

Ray shouts in agreement!

After settling into tiny motel rooms next to each other, I put on my turquoise gauze south-of-the-border style dress appropriate for our favorite food.

In the morning we board the Durango/Silverton Narrow Gauge Railroad, taking seats in the gondola car, open on both sides. We can almost touch the granite cliff we rumble past and Ray's looks at me, saying, "I love you."

After I return from the restroom, hanging onto seats, he asks, "Why do you lean to the left when you walk?"

I answer, "Because my right side's weaker."

In Silverton, the silver-boom mining town, Ray circles my waist with his strong arm, walking me in and out of souvenir shops. We eat Mexican again, deciding we'll try chili rellenos in every town to compare who makes the best. When the whistle blows we scurry through a downpour and search for seats in the enclosed car since it's chilly and my muscles ache. We snooze leaning against each other.

After I shower in the morning Ray brings me a cup of coffee, delivering it with a light kiss. This begins our deliveries to each other as "Coffee Man" and "Coffee Lady," *always* with a kiss.

On the way to a golf course Ray says, "Thanks a lot for coming with me." I *love* cheering his good shots, commiserating on the not-so-good-ones. Then we hop in his Mustang and drive toward Ouray.

I demand, "Pull over here! I want to take a picture!"

He says, "Order me around!"

I respond, grinning, "Well, I *did* warn you I'd probably ask you to pull over suddenly."

Ray lightens up after a silent period that I told myself was not my problem by saying, "I like it. You speak your mind," and he smiles.

I tell him my family camped in this area many Augusts when I was growing up, though I'm not sure how old I was. "We were on this road, The Million Dollar Highway, when it was being blasted with dynamite to widen it! You could hear this huge boom echo through the mountains as traffic piled up. One time when we left Ouray, sheep were being herded out of the high country down Main Street, which was dirt back then."

I'm transported back to happy childhood memories as I squeeze out arguments between my parents trying to surface like weeds in a resplendent garden.

After napping in the same room on separate beds in Ouray we rent a jeep, while I learn Ray has *never* driven on 4-wheel roads in the mountains! I affirm his maneuvering up the rocky, steep terrain. He thinks this is a bad road.

"You haven't *seen* 'bad' until tomorrow," I chuckle.

As I'm jostled here and there in the seat I laugh till my stomach hurts. When we stop on the promontory overlooking Ouray, Ray sets my camera on timer on a log and we sit close together on the front bumper of "Number Five," dubbed by Ray after the robot in the movie we saw on our first date. *Ah, he's a romantic.*

In the morning we get high in the canyon called Yankee Boy Basin. The double waterfall doubles itself again as it falls away from the level before it. Wildflowers burst with colorful abandon and together *we* burst into a song of praise to God, we're so overjoyed. The road is rough, and Ray admits he was afraid last night. I tell him he's a natural for taking the boulders.

Taking the number four-out-of-five difficulty road (five being the worst) up Engineer Mountain definitely challenges Ray, but I'm bounced around so much I giggle until I cry. When we return to Ouray I'm so much weaker. I feel *bad,* so I begin praying aloud with thanks for our wonderful day, with Ray joining in as we lie on respective beds.

Then I begin shivering. "Ray, I have chills up my spine from over-fatigue. If they don't go away will you rub my back to warm it?"

He says, "Sure," and starts to pray aloud for me. When my back begins to cramp, he rubs up and down my spine, soothing me. He leans over and whispers, "I love you, Jo."

"I'm going to cry. It's hard to let you see me this way."

Ray gets teary as he holds me in his arms while I whisper, "I feel as if you're sharing my burden."

He kisses my wet cheek and we shed tears together.

After changing our dusty clothes we head to the Outlaw Restaurant where we gaze into each other's eyes intently, holding hands, in the dark-wooded room.

Ray says, "I was thanking God for teaching me to have compassion through you. I feel *so alive* and glad to be learning this emotion! I've always been loving and kind at times." I sniff as Ray says, "I love you more all the time and think about how it would be to have a permanent relationship, and it seems so good."

His smile makes my heart flutter. "I don't know where this will lead, though."

I say, "I feel the same. I'm not putting expectations on you."

Ray smiles, "Thanks, I'm glad you told me that."

When we return to my room we lie on one bed next to each other to watch television, and soon we begin to kiss tenderly. Our passions aroused, we pull away from each other and say good night.

Ray slows the car as we drive east so he can watch for fish in the broad stream on the roadside. He likes to take the girls fishing. I enjoy watching his graceful casting of the fly rod. It's like a piece of the symphony created by the water bubbling over rocks, in perfect harmony.

As Ray comes back he says, "You know what?"

"What?"

"I love the way you're interested in my interests!"

I smile broadly, "I want to share them. I enjoy watching the little boy inside the expert, and I love being outside."

"What I would have missed if I let MS get in the way!"

In Glenwood Springs we border on crabbiness, then work it through with Ray asking if I think I can handle him. I say, "I think so."

Ray holds my hand. "As we jeeped I kept thinking how nice it would be to spend the rest of my life with you, married. You're such fun and have such a great outlook. But I'm afraid."

"I feel the same. Still, I think it's important to admit we have a relationship that can lead that way and work on it."

Ray agrees and says, "I love how you respond to my children."

"It's easy. I love them."

He continues, "I think you have such a great attitude to give my girls. They need someone as they get older. I can't stand to think about letting you off at your place tonight!" and I laugh.

We kiss warmly, saying, "I love you" at my door later.

In the morning Ray calls to talk about our trip, "I've thought about how God put you in my life to meet all my needs, even my strange ones. I told God *I don't need MS*. Then I realized I don't need to worry about that if God put you here. It will be in *his* hands."

I cry, "How sweet. It was so special when you shared my chills and pain."

Ray exclaims, "With all the fun and affectionate times *that was the best of all because I felt more alive and full of meaning than ever before!*"

When the girls return Lindsey sits beside me. "I love you, Jo. I missed you." I hug her and repeat the same. She asks, "Did you stay with Daddy the past two days? Are you going to stay the night?"

Ray and I both answer, "No."

Melissia's disappointed I'm leaving after dinner, but she's excited I'm meeting them at church. She says, "I wish you lived closer."

Lindsey says, "Why don't you move right in here!"

Melissia adds, "Or next door."

How do I explain to them what Ray and I think about this?

"Maybe after my apartment lease is up I can move closer. I love you, Melissia."

She says, "I love you."

Ray asks her, "Do you mind if I give Jo a kiss?" She turns up her nose.

He says, "I want to give Jo a kiss because I love her." *It's the first time he's said that to the girls!*

When I get home I record our conversation and sleepily write:

Lord, I love this man and his daughters. I can see living with them. Life would be fun and exhausting and fulfilling. Ray can be *so* hard on the girls. I want to soothe it. I see fear in their eyes while their faces contort in confusion, probably because they know he loves them so much. I wish he'd be a little less angry at times. Lord, use me to help Ray not be so harsh.

In the morning I'm welcomed warmly at Ray's church, and in the evening I have a concert here. People surround me with words of appreciation, and Anne whispers, "Ray's the nicest guy you've dated!"

Then Ray takes my hands and strokes them, saying, "It was great. I'm so proud of you. I feel like such a part of you, Jo. I was feeling vulnerable *with you.*" We both cry tears of amazement.

At home I journal—"TU Father for using me! 'May I never boast except in the cross of our Lord Jesus Christ' (Galatians 6:14)."

In a few days Ray and the girls swim at my apartment, then we go inside to barbecue.

Melissia says unexpectedly, "I love you, Jo," giving me a kiss and a hug. "And I love you!"

Ray asks, "Did you see Jo and me kiss?"

She looks up at him as he says, "I kiss Jo because I love her."

She screws up her face as I say, "And I kiss your daddy because I love him."

Melissia turns and walks to the back of my off-white couch, rubbing it with her fingers as I kneel to her level and put my arm around her shoulders.

"Melissia, when we kiss does it make you think your daddy will love you less than me?"

Her head bobs up and down as she suppresses tears.

I say, "The love we have for each other is different than the love your daddy and you have. I would *never* want to replace that love, *nor could I.* You have a special daddy and his love for you just makes me love you more, and I *do* love you *so much,* Melissia. Do you believe me?"

She turns towards me with tears escaping her eyes and says in a tiny voice, "Yes."

I ask, "Why?"

Melissia says, "Because *I* love *you,*" and we hold each other tightly.

When Ray calls later I say, "I don't know how it's been with other women in front of the girls."

He responds, "I've never told another woman I loved her, alone or in front of the girls."

I feel hugged, saying tearfully, "I'm sorry it's so hard for them, but I guess we can't avoid it since we *do* love each other."

With my impending hysterectomy and the girls' love I bare my soul:

Lord, maybe I didn't have children so Lindsey and Melissia would be so special. I don't know the reason, but I consider it *joy* to encounter the trial of my emotional state (James 1:2–4). Use it to make me more like you. Oh *do* it! I saw *Rosemary's Baby* and shouted "I'll never have a baby!"

afterwards. Did those words of a flippant teenager afraid of a movie put a curse on me? "Remember not the sins of my youth and my rebellious ways; according to your love remember me, for you are good, O Lord ... Turn to me and be gracious to me, for I am lonely and afflicted" (Psalm 25:7, 16). I grieve the loss of never having a child.

Then I sing through a flood of tears "Yet I Will Praise You" and say, "Your ways are not my ways, my God."

After Lindsey and Melissia spend a night and day with me, while I drive them home they sleep. My heart turns over with love, like a dog rolling on his back to have his tummy rubbed.

When we arrive at Ray's he says a gruff, "Hi," then continues vacuuming.

I don't know what to make of it.

Later he's warm, saying, "How did I get blessed with a woman like you?"

I tease, "I don't know, you just are!"

All of a sudden he says, "I appreciate so many things about you, but about ten percent of the time I see you as the world does, ninety percent through the eyes of Jesus."

I begin to cry.

"I feel angry then, and I don't know at whom," he confesses.

I say through sniffles, "That's normal, but you need to figure out who you're angry at. Is it because you love me, yet it's hard?"

"I don't think so. I feel MS is good for me. I don't want life to be without a challenge. I'm not dating you because I *want* a challenge. Other women would be easier. But then I would miss what you have to offer." By now Ray's tearing up, as well.

I choke out, "It hurts to talk like this and makes me afraid."

"I don't want to deny it though that would be easier." He cries, "Is there some place I can go for counseling, and the girls, too?"

God, how precious.

"I'll check into it. I don't want you to hurt, but if I didn't think I was valuable enough, I wouldn't be dating at all."

Ray snaps, "That's *my* decision, and hurt is a part of life."

Ray tells me he's grateful I accept him as he is and desire to understand him. He's feared others he dated wouldn't like him as they got to know him, since he knows problem-areas he himself doesn't like.

I respond, "Ray, last night I was so worn out I drove home crying. I journaled— 'How do I feel when Ray does so and so? I want to understand him. Give him space. Love him. Be there for him.'"

Ray says, "I appreciate that."

I continue, "I knew I loved you even more than I thought. All I need is to be loved."

His face contorts in pain. "I know that, Jo, and it's not fair because sometimes I *can't* love you, though I want to. I don't even understand what goes on inside of me. I think God will release me someday with the right kind of woman loving me. I'll change because of the belief she has in me, and I'll be able to love as I want."

"I understand that, and it just makes me want to love you more."

Quiet seems to fill the room, expanding our hearts. Ray says he's glad for the talk.

We both say, "I love you."

Ruth tells me the following day about Ray's phone conversation with her—how much he loves me; how he's almost asked me to marry him several times but feels he needs to let God be in control. Not to rush. *And to think I wrote last week if he asked I'd be engaged right now!* Ray told her it's getting harder and harder to say good-bye—he almost can't—and how ridiculous it seems to have to. He told Ruth his concerns for Lindsey's health the past few weeks, her dizziness and blackouts and how sharing it with me meant *so much.* We're thrilled it's a virus, not a brain tumor! Ruth told him she knows how concerned I've been about Lindsey—like Ruth would feel for her daughter Anna, and Ray sniffled. With all those wonderful insights, I'm still riddled with fear:

Father, you know my hidden anxieties—show me. I *fear* what the surgery will do to our relationship. *Truth*—If we have real love this surgery will grow us closer—that's exciting! And if it slows us down, that will show our weak areas. I *fear* having an exacerbation. *Truth*—You're in control and I entrust my loves and MS to you. You won't allow anything you can't use for my good and your glory. I *fear* I'll be less of a woman. *Truth*—If that's true I've always been less, since I never had children.

I've noted Ray's not-so-subtle strangeness for days, ever since we shared such joy after my concert. It's hospital-minus-one-day.

I apologize for being over-emotional and he says, "You don't need to apologize, I should. I realize I've been worried about Lindsey and I've been worried about *you*." He says, teary-eyed, "I haven't been able to love well this week," as he grasps my hand. He continues, "I don't want the MS to get worse. I might get really angry at God if he lets you have complications—*it wouldn't be fair.*"

I look into his eyes with tears in my own. "I know. Sometimes I cry, 'No more, Lord! I've had enough!' It's helped so much to talk this out with you."

I ask if I can call the girls since we four didn't pray together as he'd suggested and he answers, "Do it! This has been affecting them."

So I suggest they get on two phones, then explain that the doctors need to take out the part of me where a baby would grow because it has a problem.

Lindsey asks, "How?" and I try to explain the two options.

I ask if they've ever prayed over the phone and Lindsey says, "No, we can't hold hands."

"Well, that's okay because our hearts touch over the miles." I pray for them not to be afraid. Each of the girls' prayers is precious. I thank them and say, "I love you both."

Then Ray gets on the phone, telling me, "I love you."

I cry, "Oh, Ray, I needed to hear that so badly. I love you, too. Please come see me tomorrow night after the surgery."

I'm thrilled to awaken and find I had only the vaginal surgery with just my uterus removed. My ovaries and tubes look good now. Ray enters my room bearing two darling ceramic panda bears, and I reach out my arms for a hug.

The following evening he brings the girls, saying, "Have you noticed how Jo's eyes look like Katy's? Let's call her 'Katy-eyes'," and we all laugh. Katy's on my bed with her eyes at half-mast, and so are mine.

As they get up to leave Ray says to them, "Maybe we should put a 'y' after Jo's name because she gives so much."

How sweet!

Visitors pour in and out of my room. Even *Dad* decides to visit with Mom. I call him "Daddy" and later write—"I feel like his little girl, Lord. I love my parents so much." I'm blessed by many cards. Yet when Friday arrives and Ray leaves for San Francisco without calling, having hit golf balls the night before and not visiting, I pour out fears and misbeliefs, trying to counteract them with the truth. I try to see Ray's backing off as an opportunity to prove I still love him. I read Psalms and 68:2 jumps out at me—"God sets the lonely in families" so I write in the side column—"Given to me by God 8/14/86 while in hospital for hysterectomy." I journal:

> I'm alone with no children to love, then along come Lindsey and Melis-
> sia. Could this verse be a promise of more than the family of God I
> already belong to? I consider Ray's ignoring me as joy in this relationship
> I hold so dear to grow *me* (James 1:2–4 *again*).

When Ray calls two days later before flying home, he says he tried to call but couldn't get through. When he says, "I love you. I miss you," I respond, "I needed to hear that."

Two days later he comes to my apartment and says, "With every sunset or sunrise I thought, *Jo would be saying 'Oooo! Wow! Look at that!'* I know I wasn't enough support to you, and that wasn't fair, but I couldn't help it. Since before our trip I felt this surgery would be a turning point for us."

I gulp, "How do you feel now?"

"Like before. I love you, but I kept wondering through the week if an MS attack would hit, and didn't know how I'd react. You're adamant about someone accepting you with MS. That's a lot to ask."

I nod with a tight smile, "I have to, or I'd rather it was just me and God."

Ray nods, saying, "It's understandable, but it still takes work and time." Then he cries, "I get so frustrated! Mad at God! I try to be close to him, yet I still have this fear, these inabilities to let myself trust and let go in love. I don't understand! If it's too much for you I just need to accept that, but I can't hurry it. We've known each other four months. I feel the more I know you the easier it will be to handle my fear of MS."

I bite my lip, "Maybe it would be better for you with any number of women, not me."

"No, it would be difficult for me no matter what relationship I was in. I think about you more and more with a permanent thought in mind. I tell myself I want to date you for a long time before I make any decisions, then at times I just want it now!"

I smile knowingly, "I'm not trying to rush anything, Ray."

He says, "I consider you worth the risk even though I can't figure out what you see in me. I respect you and consider you very valuable because you love me."

"I see how beautiful you are inside. I won't retreat, but when *you* do, I'm going to call you on it! Maybe if you talk it out it will help."

He responds, "I may not want to, but I think it would be good for me."

Later, I pray, "Lord, I *do* fear. Ray's so honest about MS being difficult. I pray he goes for help *soon* because if I am wrong and he can't be there for me, I want to know."

In the morning I'm vocalizing higher and higher when an out-of-tune ring pierces my singing. I'm trying to get my voice in shape for my concert only two weeks away.

I answer, "Hello …"

A woman says, "Are you the Jo who had physical therapy in 1975 and led your PT to the Lord?"

I say in amazement, "Yes!"

"I'm Sherri, that PT! I saw your poster at my church and thought it might be you. I've remembered you *so many times* and wanted to thank you and let you know I've grown in Jesus!"

Tears fill my eyes and I'm covered with goose bumps as I ask if she'd allow me to introduce her during my concert. She readily agrees as we both decide God wants other people at Galilee to be blessed.

My heart feels like it's healing as I pray, "God, I've never had children, but Sherri reminds me that I've taken part with your Spirit in 'birthing' *your* children. I have *many* children in you, like Jessica and Sherri. Oh, thank you for this sweet reminder."

This evening is the beginning of hours and days spent with Ray, Lindsey and Melissia—hours of laughter, teasing, hugs and kisses and fun; of cuddling the girls and talks beginning with Ray's, "Hi beautiful!" We drive up Mt. Evans, and while eating in the lodge, Ray holds Melissia and I hold Lindsey.

He tells the girls, "You know what I love the most in the *whole world?* Your kisses and hugs."

Melissia says, "And Jo, too."

Ray says, "Jo's kisses are different and they're special, but yours are what I love most."

I look at him and he smiles at me. *I hurt to know I'll always be second. I guess that must be the way of a man or woman who marries and has children already. Of course they don't leave them and cleave to their new spouse. I wouldn't want that! Help me with this.*

When Ray asks later if I've had the ringing/buzzing in my ears lately, I can't even remember when it stopped! I thank him because it reminds me to be grateful.

After dinner I grasp the girls' hands and whisper, "Let's go in your room to talk about your daddy's birthday."

We sit in a circle, decide what we'd like to do, then I tell Ray, "We'll be gone a little while," kiss him, say, "I love you," and leave for the store.

Lindsey says, "If you hadn't come into our lives, Daddy wouldn't have such a nice birthday."

As Melissia looks at cards she says, "Here's one for 'Hubby.' You should get this one for Daddy."

I chuckle, "But we're not married, honey."

"I know, but you might."

I smile and ask, "Would you like that?"

Melissia nods, embarrassed, and walks behind me. As we shop I must be firm at times, thinking *I can see how it would be taxing and tiring, Lord, but you would give me what I need.* Melissia brings me a heart balloon that says, "I love you," and I say, "I love you, too, sweetie."

We take it to Ray who's not feeling well, who's actually cranky. I go to the bathroom and pray, "How do I deal with this?" Later he's warm and affectionate. I journal:

> I feel secure in our relationship, though I want to hear Ray initiate 'I love you' freely like he used to, not just follow my lead. I just had a weird fleeting thought! He might say he wants to date others and later he'll come back to decide on us. Yikes, was that to prepare and warn me of what's ahead? Or to see if I'm willing to give him up no matter how much it hurts? I hope it's not in your plan. I *will* hurt badly, but I'll accept whatever happens.

A couple days later I go to a bike shop with Ray and cringe when he says tandems are too expensive. Feelings of green envy pour over me unbidden like slime. I write:

> Would I be jealous of Ray because of his activities? I resent him because he can ride and I can't. Oh God, renew your joy in me! Jesus told Peter not to compare himself to others. When I do that I feel cheated. I need to praise you because of *who you are*—God. You know my plight about wanting to ski and ride but can't without help from others. I need to *live* 2 Corinthians 4:16–18. How petty this seems when what really matters is what is *unseen*. I must fix my eyes on heaven and you! TU for what I *do* have and what I *can* do. I have *so* much to be grateful for!

Within an hour Ray calls to tell me he saw a five-speed tandem in the paper, but it sold fast. He'll keep looking.

"I'm so ashamed, Lord. Thank you for forgiving me. Ray really does care about this love of mine. Keep reminding me of this weakness of jealousy so I *change!*"

Chapter 14

How Can This Be Good?

As Ray and I sit on my couch after seeing a movie, I ask if his parents beat him.

"Dad did when he was drunk."

My heart lurches with compassion as I say, "Severely? So you were incapacitated?"

Ray says, "A couple times."

I rub his leg. "I thought so," as I explain watching a program about adult children of alcoholics.

He whispers, "I really felt like hitting Melissia in anger when she was little and prayed a lot about it. God changed my desires and actions. I know I was expected to fall into the same pattern of my dad."

"Adults said they can't trust others because they've had so many broken promises—"

Ray cuts in, "That's right! I've been conditioned not to trust! I can't even trust God sometimes!"

"Because we expect God to be like our father," I say sadly.

Ray agrees.

Lord, show Ray he can trust you and me.

"Ray, you said you don't deserve me—why?"

"Because you're so special and accept me just as I am. I've always dreamed of that—now I have you and feel it's more than I deserve."

I tease, "So, you *have me?*"

He smiles, "Yes, I do, that's why I don't take you for granted."

Ray speaks so softly I ask, "Repeat that, please."

He says with feeling, "I *love* you."

"And *I* love *you.*"

The following evening Galilee Baptist is full as I begin my concert, weaving in songs as I share how I became a Christian; live daily with MS—a lion of fear to be caged and tamed; what I'm learning because of my divorce and my jealousy of a friend who can ride a bike alone; about my hysterectomy and grieving the loss of never having children. Then I invite Sherri on stage. She tells how she saw my poster and called. Sherri explains how I told her about Christ as she treated me with physical therapy and some of her life after that decision. The audience is once again in tears.

I say, "I didn't ask Sherri to tell this to glorify *me,* but to show how when we cry out to God for help, he answers and uses our weaknesses." The response as Sherri walks down the steps overwhelms both of us with tears of joy.

When I hear individuals' reactions later, I simply need tissues.

Ray's friend Don says, "You've helped Joyce so much. Thank you." He tells us later he thinks she's worse because she continues to work, coming home exhausted nightly, but it gives her purpose.

Missionaries from Africa want me to go there. Others want me to travel the US professionally and will refer me. *I just want what you want, God.*

Melissia leans into my hug while I sit on my stool as the music director says, "Thank you for your unique, beautiful ministry, Jo."

At dinner Ray says, "It was as if I'd never heard you before! Your voice was beautiful—I was surprised at the strength."

Lindsey puts a note in my hand:

"Dear Jo. I love you. You sure sang good for just having an operation. You know you are one of the best things that has come into my life. You're my favorite person that daddy ever dated. You're the most wonderful and faithful person I ever met. Get well soon! Love, Lindsey"

Tears well in my eyes as I hug and thank her, and Ray says, "How *sweet.*"

September 1. The girls and I excitedly bake a cake and prepare dinner while Melissia asks, "Are you glad you met Daddy?"

I exclaim, "Of course!"

Ray's like a little boy, ripping open the girls' packages. Their eyes widen with anticipation and they squeal with delight when he expresses gratitude and kisses them. He weighs my gift carefully.

His eyes sparkle. "You remembered," sighing with love as he holds his new NIV Study Bible with his name engraved on the front. He kisses and hugs me.

I give a toast, "May this be your best year yet!"

"It looks like it will be!"

September 3. I'm lying on my bed reading Psalm 40 and verse five pops out at me—"Many, O Lord my God, are the wonders you have done. The things you planned for us no one can recount to you; were I to speak and tell of them, they would be too many to declare." And I suddenly remember Ephesians 3:20 and write my prayer—"You are able to do more than I can imagine or think. *Do it Lord, I trust you!*"

I close my Bible and snuggle under the covers. Suddenly my phone rings and Ray's apologizing for waking me. After a long talk I journal:

> Lord, what a startling, sobering call. Ray's been offered two jobs in California! I've prayed because he's been dissatisfied with his job, so I said, "I'm excited for you but I'll miss you!" and Ray said, "Well, maybe we can work something out. We'll talk." I said, "I might cry, but I *am* objective, wanting what God wants." Ray told me he read some of the MS material last night. *It's an answer to my prayers, Lord! Why now?* "I love you, Ray," and he said seriously, "I love you, too, Jo." He said I must have lots of questions, but how can I say *anything* except—what do you want to do with our relationship? Could I possibly miss the opportunity of this fam-

ily being mine? Is Ray's possible move an indication of what the verses have in store?

I put down my pen, turn off the light and lie in bed with emotions bubbling up like Alka-Seltzer. I need the real thing for my upset stomach.

When he calls the next evening, Ray says he doesn't want to leave Colorado, but does want more involvement in business and an impact in people's lives, including his siblings.

"I practically raised them," he says, "but I could take the job, move, want you to come out and you might not want to. There's so much for you here."

I gulp, "I'm glad I'm a factor. A long-distance relationship would be difficult. I won't give up my love for you."

Ray says, "I agree."

I take a big breath. "I did a lot of objective, non-emotional thinking last night with the Lord. I realize you three mean so much, I wouldn't have a problem moving. And my ministry can be produced by God anywhere."

"That's right!"

"I know if I had a chance to be a part of your family I'd go."

"That's *good.*"

I lower my voice, "I didn't want to tell you for fear it would be pressure, but you brought up my being a factor."

Ray says, "I want to know your thoughts, and you mine. I asked the girls about moving to California and they said, 'Yes! Yes!'"

We agree it hasn't sunk into their minds yet. We both say, "I love you," with mine first.

When I pick up the girls, Lindsey says, "We might move to San Diego! You can't come along, unless, of course, you want to."

I chuckle, asking, "Would you like that?"

Lindsey's eyes light up as she cries, "Yes!"

I ask Melissia, and with her animated face she also says, "Yes!"

Then Lindsey adds, "I'd miss you terribly if you weren't there. We'll have to find you a place to live."

Melissia says, "You could move in with us, and maybe someday you and Daddy will get married."

I shake my head, saying, "No, Melissia, I won't move unless I am to be your daddy's wife. Do you understand?"

She says softly, "Yes."

"We love each other, but when people have been divorced, it makes it harder to marry because of fear. I prayed about it and told him I would leave *everything* to be a family with you three, I love you so much."

Lindsey says, "Well, then I guess we'd call you 'Mommy.'"

"If your daddy asks me to marry him I'll be the happiest lady in the world to be his wife and your step-mom, but it's his decision, and we shouldn't put any pressure on him."

Then Lins says, "You *need* to sing in California. There's so many people who go to church who don't know Jesus!"

I stifle a giggle because she's so astute. When Ray arrives later, as the girls sleep, I tell him what they said, and he smiles.

After Ray's company picnic, he's cold. I ask if he's feeling okay since Melissia isn't. "I have a headache," he states, but within minutes he's on the floor playing with Lindsey.

Father, how often will Ray pull back from me while he retreats into loving the girls? Should I say something?

As we pass in the hall I ask about Melissia, but he doesn't answer.

I say, "Ray," as he turns around quickly, "*Please* don't push me away."

His face contorts in pain, "Why do you think that? Maybe I just don't feel emotional."

"Maybe, but I don't think so."

He sits next to me on the couch feeling like an iceberg. I suddenly remember he was watching television earlier, when an ad about alcoholics saying we hurt the people we love the most came on, and he switched it quickly. *Did he retreat into the past? Or is his mind on other things?* As we say goodbye at my car, he hugs and kisses me lightly but doesn't say, "I love you," as I do.

I drive home crying out, "Lord, *can* he love me enough? Will I always hurt and yearn for more?"

When Ray calls the next day he isn't warm, but talks about disciplining the girls, and wanting to be careful not to break their spirits. He says, "I could, you know. I can be pretty mean when I get in a certain mood. I guess I owe you an apology. I was a real crab yesterday."

"That's okay. I love you. Did I say or do anything to contribute to it?"

"No. I get like this. I don't know what triggers it, but I have to work it through." Ray sounds frustrated. "The possible move is causing me to make decisions I don't want to make now."

"Maybe it's hard to be around me because I'm part of that, but I didn't want *us* hurt by you pulling back. You told me to tell you when I felt it."

Ray states, "Well, it didn't help!"

When Ray calls the following evening he says, "I reflected this morning, and realized I need to get my perspective back on the Lord and pray."

TU for answering my prayers!

"Sometimes I don't know why God bothers with me, but he does. His Spirit keeps working on my conscience until I know I need to talk to him."

As we share more I say, "I tried to show you I understood how difficult it is for you."

"But I didn't want to talk. You have to understand me, Jo—"

I interject, "I'm trying."

He says, "It's hard to let someone in on my problems. You just need to be quiet and be with me and I will with you."

"But I need to *talk* about mine."

"I hope to be able to someday. I want to say 'whatever you want, Lord,' but I'm not there yet, even though I know it will turn out for good. I can't emotionally accept it yet."

I say softly, "I love you. Good night." He says, "I love you, too."

Oh, TU for his desire to verbalize his love, Lord.

While Clay drives me home from the Stonecroft Ministries event the following day we share comments from those who listened. I'm exhausted and my voice shows it.

Mom says from the back seat, "If I didn't see how you help people, I would *stop* you from doing this because of how hard it is on you."

I can't believe Mom is *still* trying to exert control over me! I don't say a word, because she'll just make up some excuse for having said it, and I don't feel like having an argument, but I think *Stop me? You couldn't stop me! God has put this on my heart!*

Later I call Peg to explain how Ray said, "Let me be quiet." She agrees sometimes that's better.

"It's hard to let him have his space this week."

She says, "You're being prepared. Most don't understand that and have difficulty in marriage because spouses need it. I believe Ray can work through his emotional drawbacks because he's never really had anyone to work on it with before. He's come a long way."

The following evening Ray surprises me with an invitation to one of our favorite restaurants, Moose Hill Cantina. Melissia crawls into my booth and says, "Daddy, you love Jo thiiiisss much," as she spreads her arms through the air to behind her back.

Ray's eyes widen as he nods with his mouth agape. I squeal, "I'm right here, you guys. I'm embarrassed!"

I was literally afraid Ray would deny it or play it down because I feel so insecure!

I was vulnerable in a card saying in so many words I would go if he asked me to be his wife. When Ray is loving he's wonderful, when he's not he can be short and cranky. When he's silent I feel rejection. As Ruth says, Ray is re-evaluating our relationship. So be it, Lord. You know your plans for me. Plans for good, not bad. *Do it Lord, I trust you.*

In my next journal entry I arrow down to these words:

For sure! Ray said I was welcome to come over, so I kissed him hello, then took the girls to the grocery store. Lins said, "I asked Daddy if he's going to marry you and he said he doesn't know. He's not sure he wants to be married again." My heart dropped to my feet. I couldn't hear it beating so far away. "I love all of you so much it will hurt a lot, but your daddy may need to move away, and even be gone for months before he realizes he misses me enough to know he has courage for marriage again." Lindsey said, "I hope he decides before we move!" Both Lins and I began to cry. Back in the house Ray teased the girls and ignored me. When he left for the store, I just wanted to drive home and be alone with you, God, but when Ray returned we worked together disciplining the girls, and he sat close to me on the couch after they went to bed. When Ray kissed me all my tension melted away like chocolate warmed by the sun. *He still cares.* At my car he put his arm around me and thanked me for coming. I said, "I love you, Ray," and he said, "I love *you*." He wanted to express his love before leaving for interviews. TU God.

As I read the book *Children of Alcoholism/A Survivor's Manual*,[16] Ray jumps off every page! Since the alcoholic is unpredictable, the child has no trust for what he can expect or rely on, so fear and disappointment is his MO. Since the parents lie, family members become angry and alone without open communication. The child believes he's at fault for any violence. Neglect causes the adult child to doubt his ability to give others what they need. He feels the need to control his life, or it will fall apart. Feels like he's different than everyone else because of shame. Ray had to grow up too fast because he was responsible for siblings. He says he's taken care of people all his life. He fears me getting worse. "Oh God, if I *am* going to do so, Ray's already had his share, move him away so he doesn't have to 'take care of me.'"

Yet I still love him.

When he calls the day after he returns, he says he'll move in two weeks. The girls still want to go. I sit in shock. It's like lightning hit me and I'm immobilized. He didn't even mention *us!* "Lord, I need your overwhelming presence now to concentrate on all the upcoming ministry opportunities. Without you it's impossible to get Ray off my mind."

After prayer with Ken, Ruth, and Judie, I invite Ray over to talk. He gives me a quick hug, asks how I am, and we sit down.

I say, "I need to know what you want to do with our relationship now that you're moving in two weeks."

Ray says, "I *want* to see you, but I have lots to do and won't have much time. Beyond that, I've thought it through carefully, and I'm not ready for any greater commitment."

I don't feel surprised, I feel *dazed.* "Okay. I know you've been grateful that I accept you as you are, but one area I've brought up before that's difficult is when you pull back from me. When Peg asked how we're doing last week, I told her this one area triggers into the pain and rejection I've felt."

Ray cries, "I don't expect you to put up with me!"

"I will *not* have you move away saying Jo is just another person who rejected you! I *want* to work on this. Peg said she feels you'll be *able* to work it through. When I'm with you and the girls and it happens, I see you loving and teasing them as if I'm not there. I'm not jealous, but it's like you apparently *want* to make a distinction in showing love, and that hurts."

Amazingly, Ray nods in agreement, and I go on, "If you want us to have a possible future, now of *all times* I need you to *fight* the feelings of retreat. Maybe it sounds selfish, but I respect and value myself enough to know I have a lot of fear when you pull away. What do I base a possible future on if I feel you doing that now? The girls sense it and are confused, and they'll do the same to protect themselves."

Ray agrees once again. I sit a couple feet from him and it feels like miles.

Tears fill my eyes. "I *love* you and want to help you overcome those fears and inabilities to trust and love that I read children of alcoholics have—in order to do that I need a concerted effort from you to overcome it, *especially* now. I'm in limbo. I have feelings, too."

Ray's eyes tear up as I say, "I don't think you've ever valued anyone enough to love, love, love, even if it hurts. I may not be the one you value that much, though I *know* that doesn't mean I'm not valuable."

Ray's tears continue, "That's what I'm trying to determine, how valuable you are to me. I love you, and of everyone I've dated I'm attracted for many reasons more to you than anyone."

I ask, "Ray, are you afraid you'll have to take care of me?"

He shakes his head as his tears dry up, "No I don't fear you'll become a burden. But all you've told me is what you think, or what a book says! Until it means something to me it won't be reality. I do *not* want to work on myself now. Haven't wanted to for three weeks. Maybe it's rebellion."

"Maybe."

He goes on, "What you're saying doesn't make me want to change."

Oh, this hurts. In essence he doesn't value or love me enough to give me security now.

I blow my nose as Ray says softly, "I apologize for not meeting your needs."

I cry, "Ray, you've met *all* my needs except when you pull back! You meet needs you don't even know about just by being you!"

Ray looks awed as I say, "You'll risk with this job but not love," and as he agrees I add, "I believe God wants to do more inner healing in you."

Ray states, "I get so frustrated because I do things I don't want to!"

"All of us do, like Paul."

"I tell God *you can change me, but I guess you want me this way.*"

"I don't think he wants you this way. I think he wants you whole and *freed.* I just don't think you've accepted the key, which is love."

After we hug and give a sweet kiss to each other and Ray leaves, I write:

Maybe he feels he doesn't deserve to be happy so he sets himself up for rejection.

God, I'm confused. Why did you give me Psalm 40:5 and Ephesians 3:20, and have me share them so vulnerably with Ray only to see painful retreat? I'm telling the girls not to lose hope and maybe I shouldn't. "Though you slay me, yet I will trust you" (Job 13:15). I don't understand how they came into my life only to be gone five months later. I don't want the girls to be hurt. It was a blessing while it lasted, but seems like delicious candy offered then snatched away before I could savor it. I *will* praise you through my tears.

I'm at Ray's house, after bringing the girls home, when he calls and tells Lins to ask me to stay. Ray arrives, doesn't say, "Hi," but after a few minutes comes over to hug me and ask how my day was. He wants me to consider driving to California and fly back!

"I'm afraid if you don't go out there with us to check it out, if I just move and begin working, it will just fizzle out."

My heart sings as I ask, "I don't want that, do you?"

He answers in his tough, intense voice, "No I don't, but we have communication problems. I don't like the way you talked to me. It hurt. I know your intent, but I'm not looking for a counselor in a companion."

I say, "I had to tell you my needs because it hurts too much. How could I have communicated it differently?"

He answers, "I don't know! I don't want you reading a book to analyze why I am the way I am."

"I read it to understand and cope better with the way you are."

Ray states, "Fine. Then keep it to yourself unless I ask, 'Why do you think I do that?' I'm going to have to know you a long time before I take things like that!"

I soften my voice, "How do I let you know I'm hurt?"

"I can't promise I won't hurt you, but tell me."

I ask, "Just say, 'Ray, I'm hurting?'"

"Yes. Then give me some time. I'm not going to keep ending relationships when there are things that need to be worked out."

PTL!

I say, "I'm glad you want to work it through."

"I know you did what you did because you love me, but I didn't even want to talk to you. It may not be right, but that's the way I feel." He squeezes my hand and drops a light kiss on my mouth at my car.

I journal later—"And yet, Lord, didn't you use all of that information to *bring* Ray by your Spirit's conviction to this point of admitting he really wants to work through his pulling back?"

A few days later Ray takes me to his home and we fix dinner.

Lindsey whispers as we fold clothes, "Daddy may still ask you before—"

I interrupt, "Lins, he won't ask me before."

She looks apprehensive, saying, "Daddy isn't pulling back from you now."

I say, laughing, "No, he's not. We've had good talks," and I give her a squeeze.

She sighs, "But I'm afraid he might not decide now and he might forget about you."

I ask, "Do you think he loves me?"

"Yes!"

"Then we need to keep trusting God. Don't tell your daddy what to do. You know he doesn't like that." She laughs and agrees.

After my concert at Bear Valley Baptist, which Ray is too busy to attend, I write:

> TU Father—I felt your joy flowing through me! TU for using my pain to touch others as I said, "God is putting me back together again piece by piece as it were with his own brand of glue." The music director said before the audience, "Jo, if you're handicapped, we should all be so handicapped!" TU for using my weaknesses to prove your strength! But Lord, thank you for forgiving me for comments that hurt John and Ruth and Ken. TU for blessing me with friends who forgive and help me so much. *Never* let me take them for granted!

A few days later Ray calls, but doesn't want to talk about the dueling offers.

I say, "I love you." Ray says sweetly, "Thank you. Good night."

> I hate it—he said *thank you!* I want to throw something because this hurts so much! Yet he probably said TU because he's grateful I love him even when he needs space. God, wrap your loving arms around me. Give me peace. *Am I weird? Do I need too much reassurance of love?* "Show me your ways, O Lord …" (Psalm 25:4). I *want* to say "I love you" *unconditionally* to Ray so my integrity is intact.

Judie affirms when I call her that people *do* need space and one can give it when they feel secure in a relationship. The way I felt was understandable. I need to pray 1) for Ray to help me feel secure, and 2) to not have things "tap into my pain of the past." I pray, "Heal me of these hurts, Father. I'm as crippled as Ray."

In a few days I drive to Ray's and walk over to the girls' mom's house to meet her for the first time.

She says, "The girls really love you. That makes me feel good."

I smile and say, "I really love them." We both cry as we talk about them moving so far away.

Then Ray takes me to dinner where we talk for hours. He's letting me in on his growing excitement about his decision to move to San Diego.

As we discuss the girls I tell him, "While I was driving, Melissia teased about someone hitting us, and I said, 'I don't want to die yet.' Lins said, 'But you know where you're going.' I chuckled, 'That's right.' Melissia said, 'And you won't have to use your cool-aids anymore or do wrong and you'll be just like Jesus.'"

Ray smiles as I say, "It was so sweet, as if they've heard every word I've said."

Ray puts his hand on mine and squeezes it. He's leaving tomorrow night for a meeting and to look for a house.

After several days of journaling every possible fear and misbelief seeking to steal my peace, I counteract each with truth. Oh, but I sob. Judie says to not feel bad, it doesn't mean I'm not trusting God. She says let them flow for healing. I know she's right, for Paul said he was "sorrowful, yet always rejoicing" (2 Corinthians 6:10). I pray, "TU for her Barnabas nature. Her desire to be a friend who uplifts me along with Anne, Ruth, and others."

Ray calls finally, saying he'd like me to go with them, but he can't afford the flight back, and anyway, the car will be too full.

"Ray, will you miss me?"

He says, "*Yes, I'll miss you!* You'll write a lot, though."

I respond, "Oh, I will, huh? It's got to be reciprocated."

He says, "Yeah, or I'll call."

Lord God, I ask for mercy that Ray let me down quickly if it's over. I know you'll grow my faith. When you gave me those verses I had no idea the pain ahead. I thought it would be something *good,* but these weeks have been full of pain and I'm so weary to feel your overriding joy. I always said I wanted to be the sacrificial lamb for Ray's growth, but I hurt. Maybe we'll be married someday. I still praise you through my tears.

As I pack boxes the following evening Melissia says, "I wish you were going with us."

I whisper, "I do, too."

She says, "I'm going to miss you as much as my mommy, and that's *this much,*" spreading her arms wide.

Tears pool in the corner of my eyes, "I'm going to miss you, too, soooo much."

Lins says, "I believe I'll see you again."

I nod as tears, again, fill my eyes.

Ray tells me about siblings he wants to reconnect with, and I gently caution him to not parent them. He agrees.

I say, "You were afraid we'd fizzle. How do you feel now?"

He tilts his head, "Well, I'm a little concerned. I told you a long time back God wanted me in this relationship, and I believe that now, and if he wants it to be more, he'll work it out. I've had so many things to deal with I haven't *wanted* to deal with 'us.' That may not be right, but I just need some space and time."

"If you decide you want it to end, I want to *know.* I want closure, not fizzle or fade out."

Ray says, "I'll tell you. I care a lot about you. I just need to get my mind settled."

I say, "I'm excited for you."

"I wish you could be there with me," he responds and we say goodnight.

Father God, I just want to give you glory through my life and accept your will, but it seems unfair I need to learn through even *more* pain how much *you* mean to me. I want happiness in my life, too. I know your love is all I need. Oh God, make me believe those words I just wrote!

The next evening I drive to Ray's again. He's not happy, he's working so hard, but my intent is to help anyway.

Melissia says, "Jo, if my daddy forgot me and my mommy moved to Texas ..."

"I'd keep you! But your daddy won't forget you." We giggle as she lies on my lap while I take a breather.

Later, she tells Ray, "Daddy, if you forget me, it's okay, 'cause Jo said she'd keep me."

Ray teases me but isn't affectionate. He invites me to come over tomorrow as well.

In the morning I'm thrilled to receive several calls for ministry engagements. "I have your work to bring me joy, Lord," I pray as I drive to Ray's.

Lindsey sits on my lap after we work awhile, asking, "When will I see you again?"

Tears fill my eyes to overflowing as I say, "I don't know."

Tears escape hers, "I'll think just a couple weeks."

"I love you so much. I'd love to be a mommy to you, and it's been wonderful to have you in my life. You are *so* special."

We sit crying together and Ray doesn't interrupt. I give her and Melissia stuffed bears to remember me by.

I get down on my knees and hold Melissia in my arms as she clings to me with tears streaming down her face, and we rock to and fro.

"I love you and want to be a mommy to you *so* much. Always remember that. You have a wonderful daddy, no matter what he decides, and we have to let God tell him. *Love your daddy.* God loves you *so* much. He has good for you, remember that."

When I'm leaving she asks if she'll see me in the morning, and after I say, "No," she runs to me, hanging on, sobbing as do I.

At my car I weep in Ray's arms.

I say, "I love you, Ray," and he says, "I love you, too."

He kisses me. I cry. He tears up. We latch onto each other. He kisses me again. We embrace so hard I think I'll stop breathing. We kiss lovingly, searchingly. Rain is pelting us but I don't care.

I say, "Call me when you get there," then drive home with wracking sobs, praying I don't have an accident and hurt someone.

Chapter 15

Abandoned Again Though Determined

Ray is gone. Lindsey. Melissia. A hole as big as Texas occupies my life. I write on October 3—"God's love *requires* growth—as Paul says, I haven't yet achieved it, but I'm to run the race to become more Christ-like, more whole (1 Corinthians 9:24–27)."

When Judie calls, I tell her I've been reminding myself I also have choices.

She says, "That shows you're led of the Spirit and not just your emotions. And your willingness for 'whatever' now opens heaven's gates of blessings, because of brokenness."

My own song "You've Brought Me Through Heartache" ministers while tears flow down my cheeks.

After Ray's travel, I expect a call, but it doesn't occur. I remember Judie *and* Ray telling me James Dobson's wife broke up with him, then moved away, because he wasn't sure. Dr. Dobson had to miss her badly before realizing he loved her enough to marry.

Is that what you want Ray to discover, Lord? What of *me?* I feel so bad

about *myself!* Wait—my worth does *not* rest on a relationship but on *you*.
I am your unique, unrepeated miracle of creation. You love me as I am.
You're all I need. I want to claim your joy as you work perseverance in me
(James 1:2–4 once again!)

I'm grateful for privileges to sing and speak. A choir director says after
a women's event, "Your voice is so strong, especially for sitting down."
Grandmother commanded me, "Stand straight!" "Pull that tummy in!"
"Head high!" "Tuck in your bottom!" and I'm thankful. It helps as I sit
on a stool. And there's *always* someone in the audience with MS or who
knows someone with it. Then I share in the gymnasium of Denver Christian High.

The principal says, "I'm about to teach on First Peter, and I could preach
for months and not get across what you did!" and tears fill my eyes.

One evening I'm praying for Ray when my phone rings.

"Remember me?"

I exclaim, "Yes! Do *you* remember *me?*"

He apologizes for not reaching me. "I *did* try to call you the past few
days from work."

I say, "I've been singing. I wish you'd left a message."

I ask about the girls, and Ray answers, "Lindsey was crying last night.
She misses you and her mom so much. I told her how I cried in my foster
home not even knowing where my parents were! I remember the horrible,
lost feeling."

"I'm so glad you could share that with Lindsey."

Ray pauses and says, "I miss you."

"Oh, I miss you, too, Ray."

In the evening Lins calls and I sigh with her sweetness. Mel says in a
deep voice, "Hi, Jo, this is Melissia-bear," growling, and I giggle. Then we
exchange kisses and hugs across the miles and "I love you."

Ray says, "I'll call again, and I'll even write!"

I say, "There's mail for you at your house. I love you."

He says, "I love you, too."

I write—"Ray does *not* want 'us' to end. I feel peace that I can give him time to get settled and think. I love them. TU that I'm booked ahead for months—my life is *not* in limbo. As long as I know Ray cares I can go on with this relationship long-distance."

I send each of them cards and midweek, October 12, dial Ray's number.

He says, "I miss you," and I repeat the same as we profess our love.

Ray adds, "I have our jeep picture on the refrigerator."

Lins says, "I lay on my bed today and brushed Joe Bear and listened to your album."

Oh God, it's wonderful to know I've had an impact. I recall Melissia's draw-ing of the house with a voice coming out of it, saying, "Jo, help me know Jesus!" Tears pour as I cover a page with reasons why I love Ray.

The following afternoon I call the girls' mother and say, "You have two incredibly special daughters."

She sniffs, "Yeah, they are." We both cry. I give her my number and she thanks me for calling.

TU for the vulnerability to call and cry about missing *her* daughters. She brought them into the world—not me—yet I love them as if they were mine. Would I be a good mother, Father? I *think* so. Only let it happen if I would. I don't want to harm them in any way.

Two days later tears fall. The phone rings and the collect operator asks if I'll accept a call.

Lindsey's happy voice says, "Hi Jo!" then she chatters away.

"So you think your daddy misses me a little?"

"A lot! He talks about you all the time! He told me last night after get-ting your letter that it won't take him long to decide now. But don't tell him I told you so—he doesn't like his things to get messed up!"

I say, laughing, "I promise. I want you to know I was lying here discour-aged, and God had you call to encourage me. I miss you three so much!"

Father, you are so good!

It's still hard because Ray doesn't call all week. I *must* remember God has a bigger picture than I can see.

When he does, I say, "It's hard only talking once a week."

He states, "You wrote that. It's about all I can afford. I'll have to write."

I offer to call midweek and he says, "Sure! Love you."

I say, "I love you, too," as I start to cry.

I'm a mess! I feel like pigging out to punish myself. Get fat—it doesn't matter anyway. (I've never done that!) I feel like hitting my head or hurting myself—*What's wrong with me?* I listen to the praise tape I love and don't feel it. I want off the hook of waiting again. I'm angry with you for not answering my prayers as I want them, even if it was negative news, God. I feel a digression—how can this work without Ray being vulnerable about us? I ask your forgiveness for not trusting you. I *want* to. I hate myself for being whiney to Ray. Help me believe *you* are all I need even if I still long for them.

In a few days I call Ray. He is *not* warm.

When Lindsey gets on the phone she says, "It will be soon."

I say, "You want to encourage me, don't you?"

"Yes. I love you. Here's a kiss and a hug," and I return the same warmly.

Ray gets back on, and I remark, "You should realize this is harder for me. You're getting mail every week."

He says, "That's true. I'll have to start sending cards. Have a good week. Good night."

I shed no tears. I'm angry! He didn't want to show *any* feelings. I feel guilty for saying "should," but friends say not to feel badly, he needed to hear my feelings.

Ray calls a couple evenings later, cheerful. He says, "We're having a fun weekend, but I'm lonely. I really miss you!"

I sigh, "Oh, Ray, I miss you, too." When I tell him I tandem bicycled with Art, whom he's met, I say, "I talked about you all day."

Lindsey says, "I heard Daddy say he misses you!"

"Yes, and I'm glad!"

Melissia says, "I love you, Jo!"

After the Evergreen High Awards banquet on October 26, I write Ray—"I just got home and wish I could be a warrior-child in your arms and let you kiss away my tears— of being full of joy, overwhelmed by how God used me, the emotional exhaustion of vulnerability, nothing bad. I miss you so much, Ray ..."

I call the following evening and guess he's tired. The girls have written, yeah! Though Ray repeats he misses and loves me after I say it, there's little, if any feeling. I pray for him. Friends encourage me to give him time, and Judie affirms my growth in giving him space and how much I've grown since she met me.

But fears drag at me daily, like a flu bug refusing to give up, as weeks go by without a word. I'm going on with life, though continuing to send cards. When Ruth and I return from ministry, I erase messages I've listened to for months—"Hi beautiful, give me a call later, okay?" "I can't wait till tomorrow, can you?" and even Lindsey's touching voice. It's just too painful to hear them. "Oh, God, comfort me as only you can. You are 'close to the brokenhearted' (Psalm 35:18)."

Because I'm worried my last letter was too vulnerable, I call Peg.

She says, "If you can't share feelings, you don't have a relationship. Send a Thanksgiving card wishing them well, signed, 'Love, Jo,' without 'I wish we were together.' If Ray does call, you need to say, 'I have choices, too,' since he's not meeting your needs or keeping his word. If he sees you're going on with your life, he may come around. You can't handle this up and down—it's not good."

Peg's right. I've been saying, "I won't let this ruin my health." Last week I said, "I'm valuable and worthwhile," because I feel devalued.

A sibling tells me to go "find someone rich." *How ridiculous!*

I cry out, "God, I feel like Job again, but you know so much more than I. I will consider it joy so you can perfect me." I ache as if a bone holding my heart in place has been broken.

11/24. Well, Lord, it's over. All my hopes about Ray proved wrong. He left Lindsey and Melissia to wonder until he went out with someone else Saturday night. Ray doesn't know Lindsey phoned, crying, while I told her I loved her, how special she is, how very unique. I said through tears, "I'll never forget you and I'll always remember the wonderful times we had." She still sleeps with Joe Bear. She asked Ray if she could call weeks ago, "He said, 'Not today,' but we could call Mommy." I asked Lins if he just quit talking about me. "Yes." I told her I want all three of them to be happy and I was giving her a big hug and loved her. I said, "It's hurt so much not to hear from all of you that I prayed today you would call and you did. Thank you. Call *any* time."

Oh God, how I hurt for the girls. Heal their broken hearts. I feel anger and a loss of respect for Ray. He didn't keep his word about closure. I pray I left the girls a remembrance of a woman whose heart was so full of love for them; she wanted to be their step-mom. Who loves Jesus with all her heart, and always wants to be thankful though she has MS. I pray Ray never forgets your love shown through me.

Peg says, "I'm so sorry, Jo. You have a right to be angry. Write it in a letter. Give it a few days, re-write it, and send it if Ray doesn't call. He should hear your feelings. If he doesn't already, he'll someday regret this. You two could've really had something."

I pray, "Oh God, I hurt to have not been worth it to Ray, but I *am* worth it, aren't I? I can't see what I'm writing through my tears, but I want to give my life for others this year, this day, this moment. Use me, Lord!"

Then I throw a Christmas party for HIS MUSIC partners and others who believe in and support me. I've had trouble showing how grateful I am and needed to apologize. I don't always know how to ask for help, and yet I *depend* on people for everything.

As Christmas nears I pray for Ray and the girls, thanking God for the wonderful times we shared. I send the Christmas material that we talked about sewing and a card to all three. I know I must let them go. My heart aches as if it's been punched.

After I speak, a woman says, "I have Jesus in my life, but you have something different."

I try to explain gently that joy is trusting God to be in control, and maybe that's the difference; rejoicing in the Lord means to see things from God's perspective. *I must remind myself of this constantly, Lord. I'm soaring on the wings of an eagle as I wait on you* (Isaiah 40:31).

I've prayed over Ray's letter, and to make sure it doesn't sound vengeful, only truthful, let a few close friends read it. I share my disappointment and hurt and anger that he didn't bring closure as we promised. I say I'm sure he didn't want to hurt me, but I've wondered if I'm valuable enough to be treated with integrity ... ending, "With much pain and sadness, Jo"

After Christmas my family travels into the mountains to a conference center. They ski cross-country, but I haven't the stamina or muscles for that, so when I discover Monarch is nearby and I can ride and ski with others, I'm thrilled.

A sibling says, "It sounds like a rip-off that just because you're disabled you got a free lift ticket!"

I thought they'd be *happy* for me. Cliff, a guy who works at the center, befriends me, so we spend time together when I feel uncomfortable with my family. The following week Mom surprises me by suggesting I write my siblings.

One of you said I make a big deal about MS. When I'm with people who don't understand my limitations, I try to explain. I peer-counsel others to inform their families so they'll have support, yet after all these years I don't feel MS is acceptable to you. People need to talk, so someone shares their burden. That doesn't cause *over*-emphasis; it gives the freedom to be real, releasing stress and making the problem smaller. When I said, "I feel so and so," I heard, "Oh, everyone feels that way." Everyone does *not* feel like me. You don't know when I can't walk across a room, when I have an attack. If I have so much pain it keeps me awake at night, I'm teased about needing to sleep in as if I'm lazy. One of you said, "Come off it," when I requested help with the passing of a platter others would have gladly reached for. I've lost certain musculature I haven't been able to regain. You seem to downplay MS because I can ski downhill. I have gravity in my favor. I rest on the lift going up and can cut in most lines as an energy saver. My muscles fibrillate so I stop and rest. You don't know how badly I hurt afterwards. You don't know that I cry when I drive home from places because I'm so worn out. That I pray I won't hurt someone because my eyes become blurry, or my arms too weak to turn the wheel quickly in an emergency. That both of my feet are on the brake at a stop. I say this in all humility—I'm considered one of the best MS peer-counselors. It hurts that my own family doesn't appreciate how I try to deal with it. Some never try *anything*, yet if I do, I feel your *jealousy!* I wish we could thank God together for how well I'm doing. I love you. I hope to be a better friend and sister. I'm proud to be in this family. Love, Jo

I never hear a word from anyone about the letters.

In a few days Ruth and I fly to San Jose, California, for ten days of ministry. I fear what people at the many groups and churches will say about the MS not being miraculously healed, but instead I'm touched by love, assurances that I'm being used as I am, and desires to recommend me.

During our last two days there I feel burdened to pray for Ray and the girls, and during the flight home Ruth turns to me, saying, "I think Ray's called!"

When I push the button I'm astounded to hear Ray's voice say on January 15, three days ago, "Hi, Jo, this is Ray. I'd like to talk, and uh, I'll try back tomorrow night."

Four days later I call after praying with Judie.

I sound cheerful as I ask how they're doing.

Ray also asks about me then says, "I wanted to tell you I'm sorry for not communicating."

"Thank you."

Ray continues softly, "God keeps teaching me. I love so much about you. I don't have *any* problems with you. I just didn't want to talk. I know I hurt you. I don't blame you for feeling angry. I was afraid you wouldn't call back."

I say, "I would never want to be rude, besides, I've prayed for you."

"I didn't have the courage to tell you I needed some time alone and that it wasn't you."

Pain creeps into my voice, "I kept telling myself it wasn't me, but I couldn't be sure. Thanks for telling me."

Lindsey cries, "Hi Jo!" tells me about life, then Ray adds, "The girls miss their mom and you're not here."

I ask, "You mean they still miss me?"

"Oh yeah! They talk about you a lot. Jo, I've thought about how I appreciated our relationship. Every memory is good."

I smile. "I have good memories, too."

Ray sounds hesitant, "I wonder if you'd mind if I write and call some. If you don't want me to, I'll understand."

I breathe, "If you write, I'll write back. I'm a little cautious, though."

He says, "I bet you thought you'd never hear from me again."

I say, "Well, I prayed you'd clear this up for your sake, but you did surprise me."

"Thanks for calling back. It's good to hear your voice."

We say good-bye and I journal every word plus:

Peg, Judie, Anne and Ruth were right—Ray *did* come to regret treating me that way and losing me. I've healed so much I want to forgive. I still care. It was *wonderful* to hear his voice and know he cares for me still. Maybe you brought Cliff into my life to give me balance and keep me more relaxed about Ray, God.

When I arrive home from several days in the mountains at the center preparing excitedly for my first retreat, and seeing Cliff, Ray calls, and I realize he's tried three nights in a row! It's been ten days. I talk with the girls, giving hugs and kisses.

Joe Bear has been relegated to a shelf now just like Katy Koala. How sad. Both Lindsey and I are afraid.

"I'm glad you called."

Ray says, "I *wanted* to talk with you. I bought you a card yesterday."

We say good-bye and I pray, "You know I'm glad to hear from him and know the girls miss me, but I need him to prove his love and growth."

Then I call Peg, who confirms, "It's waiting time to see if Ray shows he cares enough."

Excitedly, I prayerfully prepare for the lifestyle evangelism talk for which Jeff and Marsha have asked me to share at their area-wide leadership conference. I love this topic because I feel like Jim Elliot, a missionary killed by the Auca Indians in Ecuador he was trying to reach. He said, "Lord, make me a crisis man, not a milepost in the way but a fork in the road, so when people meet me, they will have to decide about Christ in me."

Calls come in for radio interviews, and people are asking for a book and testimony tape! Then I get a call from Char Barnes, the pastor's wife from Grace Chapel. She's asked me to speak for their women's outreach event next Christmas for two nights. Char's so sweet. She says she really thinks Ray and I will be together someday.

In a couple days I pray, "Lord, I feel *so* weak. I could hardly walk to and from the mailbox. I feel prickly, like when a foot has gone to sleep and is awakened, with tingling in my legs constantly! And oh, the fatigue. Should I take steroids? I know you can heal me anyway. Please do."

I'm grateful as my strength returns and the symptoms subside over the next week.

Valentine's Day. I sent cards to each one, though Ray's isn't mushy, and don't hear a word, haven't for weeks. I'm sad. I'm mad. I'm *furious* Ray dropped out *again*. "Lord, help me go on." Then on March 6 I receive a sweet card from Ray. I pray, "God, I can't let Ray bounce in and out of my life like a ball that misses a court! The card melted me. I still love him, don't I?"

Skiing helps, as always. And skiing with Anne is a bucket-full of love and laughter poured into my soul with God's glorious mountains surrounding us. *TU, Lord, I can ski after the* MS *attack!*

Somehow I think Ray might call this evening, March 14, and he does. He tells me all the mistakes he's made.

I ask, "Ray, why didn't you call for five weeks?"

He says, "I've tried five times."

I respond angrily, "We talked about you leaving messages so I know you care. I want a relationship that shows I'm valuable. Why *did* you call in January besides to apologize?"

He answers, "Because you *are* valuable. I just couldn't handle a relationship."

"Ray, from my perspective you can't now. I'm not putting my life on hold. I needed to see I could trust you, and that's not happening. I want to be treated better."

"I don't blame you," he says sadly. "I guess saying I'm sorry won't make any difference."

I disclose, "I don't say this to hurt you. I wasn't looking, but someone *does* care and wants to show it."

"I'm glad for you."

"It's not good for you to come in and out of my life whenever you please. I know I care for you and the girls. It can't be good for them either. It just hurts too much."

"I know," he says. "Well, I'll let you go. Have a good week."

I pray through trembling lips, "Oh, God, solidify me with your peace. Guide Ray."

Peg says I sound healthy, no longer with the low self-esteem of hanging in because I *need* so much, which is common for women who love too much.

"If there was commitment from Ray it would be different. You could wait and work on it."

Later, I open a note from Char Barnes. Some of her ladies heard my interview on KWBI radio and were thrilled that I'm coming to speak for them in December. She writes—"You're so dear. The individual whose life eventually becomes one with yours will have to be very special indeed." *How precious, Lord. TU.*

In a month I'm shocked, scared, *and* blessed to see an envelope from Lindsey. I'm torn up because I love the girls. Deep down there's a slender hope tying up my heart that I could perhaps see growth in Ray. "Psalm 27:13 says—'I am still confident of this: I will see the goodness of my Lord in the land of the living.' I *will* wait for you. I *will* be strong and take heart."

I send Melissia's birthday card and gift, and a letter to Lindsey in early

May, asking them to tell their daddy "Hi." I hear Ray's moved north of San Diego to set up another company. He's "withdrawn and unhappy."

I cry out in prayer, "Daddy, God, I pray Ray breaks so he heals."

In a few days I pray, "Lord, am I off the wall? I feel *compelled* to write to Ray. I ask for wisdom." I recount our conversations; including him saying he was closer to God. I ask:

> "Are you at the bottom? I know you might not like to hear this, but I think you need more help. Adult Children of Alcoholics could provide that. I hurt for you and the girls … You are *so* special, Ray. You told me you believe you'd be freed to love if someone loves you in the right way, and that's somewhat true of all of us, but it puts too much responsibility on the other person. We can love fully as we let *God's love* seep into our every nook and cranny. *That* will free you to love. And when you love it is *so sweet*. I pray for you daily, at least. With his love so abundant and free, Jo."

I can't keep from praying for Ray. My heart is filling with love that I can't pour out!

> May 13: Oh God, Daddy, you are soooo good to have Char call just when I was longing for Ray. She wanted to know because she doesn't think it's over! She felt it was your will to call, relating her own experience with her husband, Paul, how they broke up, then were married only two months after they got back together.

> May 15: *Wow*, TU for your faithfulness, God! Ruth just spoke with Ray and he shared he lost the best thing—me. She told him I'd written and he could hardly wait to receive it. He wanted to call and write, but knew he'd hurt me. He said he was totally dependent on God. So Ruth and I prayed and I called Ray! I said, "I miss you," and he said, "I miss you, too. I'm so lonely. The girls are with their mom while I set up this branch. She begged to have them and they missed her so. I should've stayed there and worked on a relationship with you." I asked, "Is that what you want?" and he said, "Yes." I said, "Me, too." Ray said, "You have such quality and are

so valuable. We had something really special. I'd never find anyone like you." I teased, "Yeah, fortunately for the world there's just one of me! Ray, I've dated some since January and I *know* there's no one like you." He said, "I've wanted to call." I said, "I've sensed it." He said, "I love you, Jo. I know I hurt you and the girls a lot. I was selfish and didn't think of others' feelings." I said, "It will be hard for us long-distance." He said, "I know, but I believe God wants me in a relationship with you, so we'll just have to trust God." *PTL—Ray encouraged and exhorted me to trust you, Lord!* He said, "I need someone like you who understands me, who knows what I need and why I'm the way I am." *Hallelujah!* "The happiest days I've had were with you." I said, "Me, too." Ray said, "I intend for us to *work* on this now." I said, "Call me soon, okay?" and he said resolutely, "I *will*. I love you." And I said, "I love *you*."

In the morning Peg is exuberant. I say, "Thank you for being my pal through all this. I'll keep you informed!"

She says, "Thank *you* for letting me in on the *thrill* of seeing what's happening." Peg realizes so much benefit to what Ray's gone through to bring him to this point, even dating someone.

Ray leaves a message that very afternoon and calls in the evening!

I tell him how wonderful it is to hear his voice and, "I can't get over how great it was that *you* pointed *me* to God."

Ray thanks me for the letter, saying I was "right on," and he appreciates me vulnerably writing him.

"Ray, keep showing you care," and he says, "I will. I love you."

Two days later a card arrives in which Ray asks my forgiveness for hurting me. Tears overflow as I read, "I know that a relationship will take a lot of strength on my part, but you're worth it. I really do love and need you. Love, Ray"

In his card I write—"I forgive you, Ray. God has really been at work in you. It is so evident I'm awed ..."

Then Lindsey leaves a message and I'm thankful their mom doesn't mind me seeing them.

She says, "No problem, the girls really enjoy you."

"And you know I love them."

She says sweetly, "Yes, I know."

When I get off the phone I cry out to God, "How could *I* even imagine being a mother?" *Does every woman feel so insecure about this?*

When I pull up to the curb, the girls run to my car with huge grins. We hug and kiss often. Slurp ice cream. Buy cards for their dad and a poster for his Father's Day, which we'll decorate with pictures and expressions of love.

Lins says, "I wish Daddy had married you."

I say, "Well, we just have to pray for God's will, not ours, okay?" and they nod excitedly.

It's a difficult week, though. I haven't heard from Ray. *Is he pulling back after being vulnerable?*

When Friday arrives he says, "I've been at a convention, but I sent you a card. I'm committed to you and this relationship. I don't see myself with anyone else. I love you, Jo."

I've melted into a puddle under the chair. "I want that, too, Ray. I love you."

"I don't think there are very many people who know how to love like you do—I'm really privileged."

"I *want* to love like Jesus, though I know I don't, but I think the way to love is to not fear having you *know me.* We hold love inside because we're afraid of people knowing who we really are."

"I think you're right," Ray adds.

Daddy, God, TU for all the hurt I've had because of Ray. I think his friend is right—because Ray moved away, found out how much he loves and wants me, it will give me *more* security that he'll hang in with MS. TU that I *do* believe I can love deeply and fully because I know *your* love and acceptance so wonderfully. I've been rejected and know if it hurts I'll grow, so I'm not as afraid of being vulnerable.

While the girls and I eat pizza, Lins cries, "Daddy said you and he are getting back together!"

I smile, "Yes, we are."

Melissia says, "Daddy says he loves you. Maybe someday you'll get married."

I ask, "What do you think about that?"

She puts her finger in the air, saying profoundly, "I think it's a great deal!"

I burst out laughing and ask, "Where had you heard that?"

Melissia cries, "I just made it up!"

After many trips to the salad bar I tease, "You two must have hollow legs!" and they crack up.

I journal later—"Lord, I sense Ray might ask me to marry him when he comes here. I don't want to get my hopes up, but I'd say yes! Confirm my desires with *your wisdom*."

Though several friends are excited about Ray's growth, many, including our pastor, are doubters, telling me he should prove himself over months. I write—"TU for Ray's growth. He's reading Romans and *Why Am I Afraid to Love?*[7] He's praying you'll help him eradicate things from his childhood that cause problems."

Ray's next card says it all—"I know things will work out for us. I miss and love you a lot." He affirms my ministry, my new recording ideas, my vulnerability, and his calls increase in frequency. He says I can suggest *any-thing* to him, he knows my heart. He admits maybe he needs counseling, it helped him before. He even considers Adult Children of Alcoholics when I suggest it again. *Oh, he's growing, Lord!*

When I receive Ray's next card, I cry. He wrote the *exact same thing* in his that I said in mine, mailed at the same time—we both see how God is growing our love for one another through his will *while* we're apart. Then he calls and says he thinks about being here with me at least once an hour!

I say, "Remember the verses God gave me the night you said you had interviews in California? I wrote, 'Do it Lord, I trust you!' I couldn't figure it out but I've claimed I could trust him all year long."

Ray says, "I got the film developed of our hike last July 4. There's one of the four of us. We look like we belong together."

"*I* think so."

June 11, I learn from a specialist I have small polyps on my vocal chords. He says I can keep my next booking, but then must rest my voice and have six weeks of therapy.

"Lord, now I see why I don't have any engagements until August."

Ray encourages me to take care of myself, then says, "There are things I want to say and do, but it's just hard with the distance. I finally know what I want, and we're so far apart! 'We trust you for the timing, Lord, but can't it be any faster?'" and we both laugh.

Over lunch the next day Ruth invites me to spend the weekend with their family for my birthday. She'll pick me up for lunch on Friday, and we'll wear something pretty and feel good. I write—"Do they have something up their sleeves with Ray?"

A few days later as I drive the girls home, one of them asks me why I didn't have children, so I explain it again. Lindsey says, "But you have us!" and I say, "That's right!" She sighs, "And we don't have to share you with *anyone*."

When Ray calls he seems a bit distracted even though he begins by asking how my speaking and singing went with the polyps. He encourages me to get to bed, and we say, "I love you." I journal—"When I said, 'I'll be at Ruth's this weekend so you can call me there,' he said, 'Yeah,' as if he knew. Hmmmmm."

I'm waiting for Ruth to pick me up when she calls, so I ask, "Is everything okay? Where are you?"

She says, "Oh, I thought you were meeting me here. Sorry."

"It's alright. I'll be there as soon I can."

I weave my Mazda in between other vehicles as I speed down a busy avenue.

As I follow the maitre d' through the noonday crowd toward Ruth's table on the shaded patio, I see her stand and wave. But she isn't alone. Next to her at the table is a pair of hairy, strong forearms holding up a newspaper.

I know those arms! Ruth is grinning and looks like she's eaten a canary. I rush toward the table and the newspaper slowly lowers to reveal Ray's broad, engaging smile. He stands, and I fall into his embrace as we kiss.

"You two," I scold, giddily.

The crowd around us claps and cheers! Ruth slips away from our table as Ray gives me a surprise birthday lunch I'll never forget. People seated around us smile and whisper. I glow. Rich seafood crepes add to the glorious richness of the moment as Ray explains how they cooked up the plan to get me there.

He says, "You haven't changed a bit. You're still beautiful."

Following a lovely afternoon lounging by my pool, sharing memories, Ray takes me to Moose Hill Cantina for dinner. Romantic Mariachi music serenades while we order our favorite, steaming, chile rellenos with oozing cheese. Ray tenderly reaches for my hand across the table.

"I came to surprise you for your birthday, but I also want to ask you something."

His thumb gently strokes the back of my hand. He pauses and gazes lovingly into my eyes. My heart pounds loud enough for all to hear.

"I know we've both been scared of commitment, but will you marry me? You can have time to think about it if you want."

My eyes mist over as I squeeze Ray's hand. "I don't need to think about it. Yes!"

I look into his eyes sparkling like mine with tears of joy, as he leans over to kiss me.

After dinner we pick up the girls, another part of "the plan," and take them to a McDonald's.

Ray says, "Girls, I've asked Jo to marry me. Would you like her to be your new step-mom?"

Their eyes light up as they cry in unison, "Yes!"

Then we four drive to the Peters' house where Ken looks like Ruth. He teases, "Well, were you surprised?"

I say, laughing, "Yes!" without admitting I'd been curious, and they throw me a wonderful birthday party to top off the day.

The four of us spend all weekend together. On Sunday we attend church, already looking like a family. As I take Ray to the airport, we pray to be in God's will, to know *his* timing. We kiss goodbye and declare our love. *I'm engaged to Ray!*

At midnight I leave a message for Ray, "If you're thinking what I'm thinking, call and wake me up! *Why are we waiting? I want to be with you NOW!*"

When Ray calls at 1:00 a.m. I'm so sleepy I walk into the closet and can't find my way out, while trying to locate my phone.

Ray says, "I thought you might call. *I've been thinking the same thing! I want you here!*"

Chapter 16

A Terrifyingly Sweet Beginning

The next two weeks are a blur because Ray and I decide upon July 3 for our wedding in the Peters' backyard that so appropriately seems like the mountains.

Mama cries tears of happiness, saying, "My prayers are being answered. The past few years have been hard for you. Ron's felt very guilty."

"I haven't wanted him to."

She says, "I know. It's not your fault."

When I reach Ron to notify him to not send any more payments, I say, "I hope seeing God work so much goodness in my life can help *you* be happy."

He answers softly, "Thank you. I've been praying you'd be happy."

As I pick the girls up at their mom's to shop for dresses, I say, "You know I really love the girls."

"And they love you," she responds. "That means a lot."

"I love you, Jo," Melissia says, hugging me.

I'm hugging her back while saying, "I've always wanted the very best for all of them."

Their mom and I are both crying as she says, "And they're getting the very best." We hold each other tightly.

"Thank you so much. I'll never try to usurp their love for you, and you'll always be their mother."

She says, "That's good, Jo, I appreciate that."

During a call Ray says, "I hope people know *God* put us together—he should get the glory. I was riding my bike up a canyon listening to your recording through my headphones and heard God say, *'Marry Jo.'* The enemy will attack us but we'll have a great marriage because it's based on God."

Now it's our wedding day and I feel bluer than the sky—Ray's withdrawn! I journal—"God, *should* I marry Ray? *Truth*—Ray *does* love me."

I say, "I'm wrenched with fear but I love and believe in you," and he responds by *showing* he loves me.

Late in the afternoon Ray, Lindsey, Melissia and I stand in a circle. Our pastor begins, and on cue, I quietly sing accappella the first two lines of "Household of Faith"[18] holding Ray's hands. Then I let go of his and take the girls' so we four hold hands while I complete the song about when trouble comes our faith will keep us strong as we build a *home.* Everyone is surprised I'm singing due to the polyps. Ray kisses me boldly after our vows, then thanks God for me before all. It's the most precious ceremony I've been to and it's *mine.*

We leave the girls with their mom and head towards Ouray, but my lover pulls into his turtle shell off and on, and I can't be giddy.

"Ray, I'm scared."

He replies, "I don't know what I'm afraid of, but don't give up on me."

I say tearfully, "I won't."

When we near my new home, I exclaim, "It's beautiful here!"

We hug and kiss when he arrives from work the first evening as he sighs, "Oh, it's nice to have you to come home to!"

After dinner he says he felt bad for sending the girls to their mom's while he set up the business. This big strong man lets me hold him as he cries, "I swore I'd *never* leave the girls or let them down because I sobbed for my mother in the foster homes. I couldn't understand why I was there. Now I do. There was little food in the house. Sometimes I fixed all six of us catsup sandwiches. The people from social services just took us away. Mom *never* came to visit."

I sniff back tears as he says, "I want to be freed of the pain."

"I'm here for you."

Ray straightens. "I'm *so* glad I could talk to you—a weight lifted off me. I've *never* told that before."

Another evening Ray's eyes fill when we hear on TV it's never too late for a father to give his son the blessing of "I love you." Ray's dad died when he was thirteen, in a foster home.

I tearfully hold Ray as we both say, "I love you."

When we visit Ray's friends, he explains how I want to get all I can out of life despite MS. "We're going to get a tandem, and Jo skis as well. She's a gospel singer."

I'm tickled as Ray says, "I'm *proud* of you."

But when we get home I feel inept. He questions the calls I made. *Am I stupid?*

Then he barks, "Why *can't* you ride a bike alone?"

I'm stunned. *He can see my lack of balance!*

The following day I push the answering machine to hear, "Hi beautiful. Give me a call …" Ray apologizes, which isn't easy. He admits as a perfectionist it's hard to accept others.

I tease, "God's using me to break that in you," and he laughs.

After walking, using my cool-aids, I journal—"TU Lord, I can walk, even with pain—I'm not paralyzed or numb. TU I can smell and see lush vegetation. TU for speaking to my heart, *'I love you, Child.'* When Ray is hard on me help me speak up."

The owner of a recording studio I've been researching invites me to sing a solo in his church, and I'm thrilled to have a strong, clear voice. After prayer with Ray and Clay, who wants to continue helping with HIS MUSIC, we decide I'll record here. When Clay informs me Family Radio Network International Headquarters requested albums for *all* their affiliate stations I write—"PTL, it will be played across the U.S., West Indies and other parts of the world via short wave radio! God, use it!"

One evening I ask Ray if I can sit next to him—I've already seen what happens when I just do.

He says, "I guess you know closeness scares me sometimes."

I nod as he adds, "I keep expecting you to leave. Reject me. So I do things to push you away."

Tears pool in my eyes as I admit, "And it hurts so much I don't know what to do."

He says, "I'm so messed up I don't know what to tell you."

Almost daily I defend myself to Ray's belligerent interrogations regarding the grocery bill, a store location, a phone number.

God, I feel *frightened* by Ray's attacking tone. I try to remember he loves me, but it's difficult. I feel unattractive when he retreats. I need to remind myself daily I'm your creation. TU for my lover, my friend, Ray; for the trial of adjusting to his communication; for missing friends; TU for …
A preacher said, "We'll always rise to the level of our inadequacy—God planned it that way." I pray we both learn to depend on you.

This evening the cool ocean breeze suddenly halts and warm stillness hangs forebodingly in the air. Ray slowly lays the open book *Healing of Memories*[19] on his chest, closing his eyes.

"I was just remembering my mother crying out for me to protect her from my dad's fists. I ran into their room. Stood between her and him. He hit me instead."

Tears trickle out of the corners of Ray's eyes as I kneel beside the couch and put my face next to his, saying, "I'm *so* sorry."

We cry together, then kiss.

It's August and we fly off—Ray to the East Coast for business and I to give concerts in Colorado. I show pictures of our wedding to Mama and discover Ron surprised them with his fiancée at the family reunion. It's great to see friends and family, but I realize part of me is missing without Ray.

Our first evening together in sixteen days is *wonderful*. Then the girls arrive and hugs and kisses abound.

Melissia says, "You're a good mommy and I like your suppers! I love you thiiisss much!" running to me with her arms back.

I grin, saying, "I love you more 'cause I'm bigger."

She teases, "Well, I've loved you *longer* 'cause Daddy talked about you constantly!"

Then in bed, after Ray's emotional distance, he says, "I don't like that you're talking to me like I'm a child."

I wince and cry, "Please tell me when I do it, so I'm aware."

He says, "It's not often," but I pray, *change me, Lord!*

Two days later Ray becomes angry. Later, I journal:

We tried to work it through, asking the girls' forgiveness for frightening them. I cried, *God, help us make them secure!* I feel *rage* when Ray isn't kind, ignoring me. When he returns to his relaxed self after I've fought to be normal—not taking responsibility for *his* behavior—he's warm and *I'm* hurt and angry. After church, at Roene and Larry Lettow's over dinner, Melissia said, "I don't think Jo will ever be Daddy's ex-wife." I fought tears. I feel like crying *a lot.*

The day before school begins the girls and I are talking about how their daddy and I eventually got married.

Lins says, "I wanted a mom to be at home. I want to be a little girl with a mommy. It's hard for a daddy to raise daughters."

"I'm *privileged* to be a mom to you."

She stutters, "I mean—do you *want* us to call you that? We didn't know."

I grin, "Of *course*—if you want to!"

Both girls cry happily, "Then we'll call you Mom!"

They're proud for me to walk to their classrooms, standing in line with them, Melissia being first. She leans in to my body affectionately. My heart swells. I love hearing about their day. We decide they must take turns about who goes first, otherwise they argue, they're so excited to talk to me.

Tonight I ask Ray, "Do you realize you've walked away each time I've told you I love you?"

He answers, "Yes. I haven't *felt* like saying it because I feel pressured—you're acting insecure."

Tears flow as I say, "I tell myself the truth—how special I am to God, but I still fear."

Ray says, "I liked how secure you were." I sob, "Well that makes me feel terrible, but I can't help it." Ray strokes my back, saying, "We're getting there."

I'm comforted when Ray walks with me on the beach the following afternoon. As the girls frolic in the ocean foam we fall into step and he's my coolest aid. Melissia prayed this morning, "God, I hope you'll be happy as we give you praise at church and I hope you give us a happy day at the beach." I'm *sure* God is happy and I know *I* am. It reminds me to pray daily:

> Love unconditionally, Jo. Not so Ray will be loving, but because *you loved me*, God (1 John 4:7). Give me a wonderful sense of who I am in you, so I'm a confident wife and mother who commands respect—no matter *how* Ray treats me. Father, TU for this trial by fire.

Twice the following day Ray says, "I love you" in the girls' presence, but Melissia exhibits deep fears. One day she's so afraid I won't find my way home from school she cries. When she can't locate me in the grocery store, she weeps, saying, "I was afraid someone had stolen you!"

Then suddenly, she runs upstairs to her bed sobbing, "I want Mommy!"

God, what do I say and do? In a fetal position, Mel wails from the depths of her soul. I say, "She's not here, she's in Colorado, sweetie. I'm sorry."

Melissia cries as if she doesn't hear me, "Where's my mommy? Where'd she go?"

"She's not here, Melissia. She loves you. She always will. I'm here. I might need to go away on trips, but I'll always come home. I love you."

When Melissia settles down she says, "I love you," as she grasps me. Then she cries off and on. I feel totally drained when Melissia finally curls up in my arms as Lindsey watches everything.

In a few days, after I spill sauce from the grill on the patio, Ray frantically cleans it up while I go to pieces. *I just can't measure up.*

It hurt when Ray said, "You're different than the woman I fell in love with"—*just like Ron.* I agreed I *am* different because I *won't* accept the pullbacks he committed to change. He half-nodded. I said I don't think he's used to someone caring like I do—he admitted it. His need for control and his desires to be foremost confuse me. He nodded again. How do I have the self-assurance I had as a single when I risk rejection just *sitting* next to him? He said, "I *do* love you." If it weren't for you, God, I'd return to my safe friends. I'm *afraid* of Ray. Mighty Comforter, help, I feel like *coming out of my skin!* I have a retreat to prepare for. I need to live what I'll teach—that praise changes my attitude no matter what the circumstances. That joy is *knowing* you're in control, not being happy. That you *are* faithful to bring me through *anything*.

In the morning Ray says, "I'm sorry for hurting you by saying you're different. I should've said *our relationship* is different. I'm committed to this marriage and I'm *going* to make it work. We'll have what we want, and I love you very, very much."

Lord, TU! After we discuss various issues I write—"When I feel secure in Ray's love and acceptance, I'm not defensive!"

But the following evening I state, "Your aggressiveness has eaten away at me all day, and next time I hope to have enough courage to yell back, to keep you from running over me!"

He shouts, "Good for you!" as I whirl around to flee upstairs to relax my aching muscles.

After praying I return to say, "I was wrong. I love you as you are, but I don't want to become aggressive just to live with you. Instead, I'm going to say, 'I don't like the way you communicated that, please rephrase it so I can respond correctly!'"

I weave my way to the kitchen, inhaling a huge breath to calm my booming heart. Ray follows and lays his head on my shoulder, saying, "I really appreciate you telling me your feelings. I love you. You're a *good* woman."

I stand and cry in his arms as he kisses me.

Surely I can sit next to him now, but as I do I feel Ray's body solidify. It's as if the soft love became steel. I leave as Melissia snuggles into Ray and he tickles and hugs her.

In bed I say, "It hurts so much to scoot over to you for a warm fuzzy and you're unresponsive. Then to have the girls come—and you *know* I don't feel resentment—and you love all over them."

Ray's quiet. Eventually he says, "Thank you for telling me. I need some space to think it through."

The next evening Lins makes a toast with her Jell-O parfait, "To this family *God* put together," and we all smile.

Ray says, "Whatever Jo tells you to do, do it."

I add, "I may make mistakes, but I'll try."

Later, I tuck the girls in, singing them one of my songs, and they tell me they don't want me to go away to speak.

"How will we go to sleep without you?" Mel asks.

I answer, "Well, I'll just have to call and tell you goodnight!" and they grin.

Lindsey's crying, so I ask, "Are you sad?"

She answers, "No, it's just that I love you so much!"

I squeeze her, then go downstairs smiling from my head to my toes.

During our family-time the following evening I have Lins read Psalm 40:1–11, then explain God's produced in my life what these verses say, and I have to tell others. I ask Mel to read Psalm 23 and say, "God will prove his faithfulness with my return!"

As I pack, they cry again. I reiterate, "I'm coming back."

Mel asks, "Is this the last time you have to go?"

I say gently with a hug, "No."

Ray says he'll miss me and to all I say, "I wouldn't miss being with my family for *anything*." And I call every night I'm away.

When I arrive at the airport gate, Melissia grabs me, "Hi Mommy!" as Ray teases, "We had an agreement—I get the first hug!"

I say, "I was afraid you three wouldn't need me."

Ray beams with love, "We missed you!" A huge computer banner hangs on our wall yelling, "Welcome Home, Mom," and I laugh.

As Ray holds me, saying, "*Now* our family is complete," I sniff back tears.

The girls asked me to help them call me "Mom" early on, so I ask Lindsey if she wants me to remind her.

"Yes! Tell me so I change."

When she and Ray leave on an errand Melissia says, "I love you, Mommy."

Tears fill my eyes and she says, "Don't cry, Mommy."

I sniff, "I just want to be a good mommy."

She says, "You're a *great* mommy. I love you *just* the way you are. Don't be *anybody* else."

Doesn't her need to assure me indicate my insecurity? My role is tough. I ask God's forgiveness and the girls' when I sound critical. *I want to be different than Mom and Grandmother, Lord. Keep me listening and loving and caring even when I'm so exhausted I have MS brain fog. Especially when I swat them, like I did Melissia for the first time. Should I even do that? I know I'm never to discipline when angry, but it's hard, and I'm to always express love afterwards.*

One evening I ask *Ray's* forgiveness.

He begrudgingly says, "Apology accepted," and sulks.

"Can I have a forgiveness hug?" I ask.

He states, "Yes," but barely touches me. I sense God's forgiveness but not Ray's. "I don't *feel* forgiven—"

Ray cuts me off with incredible sharpness, "Look, I just need time to work it through!"

I cry, "Work through what—*forgiveness?*"

I shake with fear as I run upstairs. *He could've hit me, he was so angry. He wouldn't, surely.*

I find myself later in a corner of the bedroom in a fetal position, sobbing, rocking myself to and fro! When he comes to bed, I can't lie next to an icy, unforgiving man I love. I take my pillow to the couch but can't sleep, so I get up to write:

When I was dead in sin you raised me up and seated me in the heavenlies with Christ Jesus (Ephesians 2:6). I didn't deserve it. TU for allowing this garbage to come up—fear, hurt, rejection—I'm discovering the real me. The intensity of this adversity will only be within the bounds of what will make us into your people!

When Ray asks me to lunch he says, "You're *forgiven,* okay?"

"I'm genuinely sorry you felt badgered."

He responds angrily, "If you push me that's how I'll react! That's my character. I don't like the way you talk to me. It seems like an attack."

"I'm frustrated. I use 'I feel,' 'I think,' 'I need,' but you're defensive. We're both insecure."

He sighs, "I need to re-read *Caring Enough to Confront.*"[20]

I'm excited to find a used tandem in the want ads, so we take a fun, short ride. It's just what we needed. Later, in bed Ray holds my hand, asking, "What do you love most about me?"

"How you want to be like God, and your strength—though it's the greatest source of frustration."

Ray says, "Yeah, I have to keep killing my pride."

I continue, "I love the little things you do to show you love me, plus the way God uses you to mold me. How 'bout you?"

"I love your kindness, your forgiveness, your understanding."

I journal—"You *are* producing in me the very things I want most, though I fail so often!"

Before Ray leaves town for work I slip a card in his suitcase. I plan that every time he travels, he'll have a card to open—sometimes funny, sometimes sexy, sometimes mushy, about missing him, wanting him, loving him.

While the girls and I are alone we get along well. They bring up their fear when he quit calling me, then Melissia cries, "But Daddy chose you and he'll never get a divorce!"

I state, "That's *right.*"

She grins. "I ask Daddy a thousand times if he's happy and he says, 'You'd better believe it!'" and I smile inside out.

Roene Lettow drawls, "When I saw your hand lifted in the air to God while you sang at church I thought, *this is someone I can serve.*"

She suggests me to the local Stonecroft Ministries and a Colorado rep makes sure I'm known as an approved speaker. I invite two neighbors to attend my first outreach luncheon. The response overwhelms me, and Roene's help, kindness, and encouragement remind me fondly of Ruth.

One day I tell Ray I'm content in California and he agrees, adding, "I realized yesterday there's not only a special feeling in my heart for the girls, there is for you, too." I'm crying as he continues, sniffling, "I mean it's natural with the girls, we've been through a lot and they're my children, but I feel you and I are *one.* That's a real breakthrough."

"Oh, Ray, thank you for telling me. You made my day. I love you!"

October 19, 1987. Melissia snuggles up to me on the loveseat saying, "I wrote in my 'Me Book'—Mommy is singing and Daddy is playing his guitar."

She looks happy. Suddenly she breaks into tears, crying, "I don't want to grow up!"

I ask, "Why?"

"Cause when I do you'll all have to die. Will I see you in heaven?"

I say, "I hope so. I'll be there." I hesitate. Ray and I have talked about this moment.

He asks Mel, "Would you like to all be in heaven together? Would you like to ask Jesus to forgive your sins and become a Christian?"

She sighs, "*Yes,*" and prays with Ray.

Mel tells Lins and by the evening's end she, too, knows she'll be in heaven with us. We're *all* excited.

A few nights later Ray tells Melissia, "Why don't you have Mommy take you ..."

It's the first time he's called me that to them!

In bed he says, "I'm really impressed with how much the girls love and respect you."

I say through tears, "I love them so much. It's a privilege."

"It's a privilege for *them.*"

Then he says he wants to go to counseling together, but not drag up his past. *How can he dissemble his anger without that? It's stored up in reserve, ready to set off like a bomb by the flick of a switch!*

I've been suggesting we need a date, having read to Ray from a couple sources the primary relationship in a family needs to be the husband and wife or a couple courts disaster. It's been a month. I ask again and he says, "Soon."

I plead hysterically, "*We need time alone.*"

Ray yells, "There's no *need* for that. You're upsetting the girls!"

Utterly ashamed, I apologize, but both say, "You're not upsetting us."

Ray responds, "We love each other very much," as he hugs me to them in a four-person-hug.

Alone, I cry, "*God, what's wrong with me? I've never gone off the deep end like that before!*"

When we have that date, after I leave lipstick-kiss-imprints on the girls' cheeks, we watch a hilarious movie, then talk. Ray tells me he's not going to give up until he's straightened out.

"When I feel insecure I hate myself," I say with a sigh.

He urges, "But I'm not *making* you feel secure. I can have loving thoughts about you all day, then walk in the door and *something* goes off inside me and I'm afraid. I walked in tonight, praying, 'Lord, I love this woman deeply. Help me to keep from causing a bad evening because of my past.'"

In the midst of all the ups and downs I'm recording. When the producer attempts to tape my testimony I begin, "I had a happy childhood. Stop. That doesn't sound right, let me try again."

Then again. And again. All of a sudden the equipment breaks down and we have to reschedule!

When Melissia speaks to her mom next time, referring to me as "Mommy," she hears, "So you call her that now?" The girls feel awful.

"It's hard for your mommy," I say, "but you have a right to call me whatever you want. She'll grow to understand." Ray and I read in a step-parenting book that children should make the choice and *all* parents should support them.

Lindsey calls me "Jo" and I feel terrible for her guilt. Then on Sunday she asks her mom to mail another picture since they can't find the one she sent.

Her mom says, "Maybe somebody didn't want it up," meaning *me*. I wouldn't *dream* of hiding her photo! I write a letter to encourage her, but also explain I would *never* do what she implied.

As Lindsey struggles with what to call me I say, "Girls, *whatever* you want to call me is fine."

Then Lindsey calls her mom. "Mommy, I want to call Jo 'Mom.'"

She answers, "It's okay. I understand. It just hurt me at first. I have to get used to it."

A week later Lindsey smiles, "You know, Mommy? It's so comfortable and easy to say that. I'd have a really hard time calling you Jo—and I won't need to anyway!"

During our next argument Ray accuses me of having a vindictive spirit. *God, do I?* He says I'm hopeless. *Just as Ron accused—I'm* not *hopeless!* Ray comes through the doorway, encircling me in his arms, saying he should've forgiven me sooner; he has a lot of anger inside.

"Those things weren't true. I said them to hurt you."

I utter, "You *wanted* to hurt me?"

"That's the only way I know—hurt back when I'm hurt."

In bed Ray prays, "Lord, help me know how to make this relationship better. Forgive me for being angry, but I'm so frustrated. I cry out to be freed!"

Our first Thanksgiving begins happily as I help Lins make a pie and Mel a salad.

TU for patience though I was exhausted, Lord. Lindsey proudly used her bun-warmer made in Girl Scouts, inscribed, "The Franz Family." Then Ray got in a black mood and while everyone slept I wept on the bathroom floor. God, I don't want to be treated this way. Did I make a mistake marrying Ray? He doesn't want to heal badly enough. Intentionally hurts me instead. I sing my song "He Knows" because you *do* know my hurt, my fear, my suffering. I thank and praise you, and implore you for more grace.

Ray sweetens up, then he's unforgiving again. I panic. I cannot *stand* to lie next to him sleeping peacefully after he says, "I want to forgive. I'm working on it." I go to the girls' room and tell them not to worry, we'll work it out, but I'm fearful our arguments affect them. I scramble to the couch but sleep fitfully.

The next evening Ray apologizes with pain etching his face. "I couldn't sleep because I was afraid you'd give up on me."

We hold each other tightly as I remind him I will *never, ever* give up.

He prays, "Lord, I've given you permission to do *whatever* to make me like you. I want that more than anything. Thank you that you won't give up on me."

Chapter 17

Horror Reveals Itself Thanks to Ray

As I packed this time, the girls were confident I would return. I'm still glad I turned down engagements out-of-state—our family needs time *together,* not apart.

Ray tells me long-distance, "You took a big risk marrying me." I agree. He continues, "I'm so glad you're an encourager who wants to grow and willingly takes responsibility for yourself." I give kisses and hugs to the girls and say, "I love you," to all three.

When I asked my friend, Char Barnes, the women's ministry director of Grace Chapel, if Mom could attend one of the outreach banquets, she gently reminded me there would be one less seat for an invited person who doesn't know Christ. I felt badly, but I *need* Mom to hear me again. *Am I still looking for her approval?*

At home, a wall-spanning banner with a lady skier on either end of "We missed you a lot!" welcomes me. I feel loved, but I'm an emotional wreck, asking the girls' forgiveness for my crabbiness.

Ray arrives from work lashing out at me for running out of laundry detergent. I ask him to please say it differently so I won't be defensive. He states I haven't grown at all. That I "never" do this and "always" do that.

I erupt in tears. As fast as Ray exploded, he's quiet. He holds me tightly while he asks God's forgiveness and mine.

Ray pleads, "I was angry at *God* for not changing my anger at *you*."

"But Ray, God *is* changing us—you took responsibility *immediately*."

His smile spreads slowly as a headlight illuminates truth.

"*Thank you* for being strong enough to stand up to me. For asking me to please stop speaking to you that way."

We apologize to the girls for scaring them, saying we worked it out and love each other, then Ray says tearfully, "I can't change without God's help. I need him so much."

Ray's gone when the girls' mother calls, telling Lindsey it hurts her to hear they're still calling me, "Mommy." She says it's not their fault, but *mine*. I must've made them feel they *had* to, even though I didn't ask. She tells them to be sure they know they have only *one* mom. She does admit, though, it's her fault they aren't with her now. (Ray tells me long-distance, "That's *growth* for her.")

I sigh, "*Whatever* you feel like doing is fine." I ask Lins, "Do you think it would be best for me to *tell* you not to call me mom? What do *you* want apart from everyone else's feelings, Lins?"

She says tearfully, "Call you 'Mom,' too."

I write another note to their mother—"I'm sorry my letter hurt you. I wanted us to have a good relationship. I ask you to forgive me. Love, Jo"

Then Lins and I argue and she says, "I want to call Mommy." Ray tells her that's *not* going to happen after arguments. He says, "She should mind you, but you don't have to do all the disciplining—we'll work together."

Lindsey later apologizes and we hug. When the girls' mom calls in a few days she asks Lins to tell me, "Hello and Merry Christmas." *Oh Lord, TU for leading me to write her.*

In January, when Ray asks how I'm doing, I answer, "My emotions go whammy and I feel like disintegrating, like hiding. I don't know if it's hormones, but I'm *scared*."

As I cry, tears roll off my face onto his shoulder while he strokes my back. Ray tells me he felt God's love as a father for the *first* time one day last week, asking me to pray he'll experience that more. Then he admits he gets angry to protect himself from being vulnerable because of lack of trust, so I get hurt. He's afraid he's already caused the girls damage and hopes to turn it around.

"I never dealt with *any*thing until a year ago and was fine."

I say softly, "Lindsey told me when we were dating you would click into moods for no apparent reason."

He's glad I told him. He had *no* idea.

When Melissia asks me to go whale watching with her class, we snuggle close, giggle and cheer when we see a humpback whale, but things aren't always such fun. One day when I discipline the girls, I see in my mind's eye *smashing* them into the wall. I'm horrified. I would *never* do that. A vague recollection comes to me …

Rhonda's twinkling blue eyes look up at me mischievously as I say firmly, standing above her in the disheveled living room with my hands on my waist, "Clean up this mess."

I yell, "Mom and Dad put *me* in charge! I'll *make* you do it."

I slam my fist in the middle of her back as hard as I can, knocking the wind out of her. Anger quickly dissipates into sorrow.

"Are you alright? I love you, Rhonda. I get so mad sometimes."

I cry as I comfort my sister. "I'm so sorry. I was just afraid I would get in trouble."

I feel a boiling cauldron of rage inside me. God, don't *ever* let me hurt the girls. Calm me. Out of my innermost thoughts come filthy swear words I hardly used as a rebellious teenager. *Why, Lord?* I'm scared. Cleanse me. I stretch my hands upwards. I sense your nail-pierced hands reaching to mine to hold me, to lift me above physical pain and emotional upheaval and give me peace. I hear in my spirit—"*Come to me, Jo, who is heavy laden and I will give you rest. I love you.*" TU Jesus.

The next time *Ray's* angry, he blurts out vehemently, "You don't care about our home," because dishes are in the sink. The argument escalates out of control.

I write—"Why am I trapped by defensiveness, Lord? It's in relating to *Ray* that I need approval and love. I hear—'*You are my child. I love you. We'll overcome this by my Spirit. Don't be discouraged or afraid. That is from the enemy.*'"

Eventually Ray apologizes and prays to not be so blaming and attacking.

I beg, "I'm overwhelmed. We need to keep our pre-marital commitment to our pastor, and see a Christian counselor."

He states, "Okay, but if I don't like him *I won't go back.*"

As we sit together on a couch in a warmly decorated office, facing the counselor, the former pastor's easy smile relaxes me when he asks why we came.

Ray states, "I communicate in a controlling way that's hard to accept, causing hurt."

I add, "And I react defensively."

After we continue, he says, "A person like you, Ray, expects certain things from people who then feel guilty, or like failures."

With tears building, I say, "That's *exactly* how I feel!"

As we leave Ray says, "I'd better see results next session, because I'm *not* going to spend money messing around!"

When I schedule our next appointment I'm encouraged to continue standing up to Ray. During that session Ray explains we couldn't have a better step-family situation. He says, "It was important the girls look at someone I married as a mom, and they do. They love Jo so much."

Our counselor asks if I can discipline them, and we say, "Yes." He's glad.

Later, I'm tearful as Ray prays, "Thank you for Jo, for all she does for me. For the good mother she is. For this relationship. Help me encourage her."

TU God for Ray.

When the counselor asks about our marriage the next week I say, "Ray's un-forgiveness in bed reminds me so much of Ron. I'm angrier than I've *ever* been. It scares me."

Ray says, "She *is* becoming angrier, and it's not in her nature."

He asks if we think being angry is wrong.

Ray says, "No," with my adding, "It's a God-given emotion, but I'm mishandling it! I fear arguing because of my folks."

Ray adds, "I'm so frustrated. I feel discounted because Jo justifies her actions or gets defensive. How *should* I say things?"

He answers, "Don't use questions 'Why aren't you _____?', 'Isn't that__ ___?', 'Don't you think _____?', and 'Why don't you _____?' because these sound attacking."

Ray barks, "How long will it take me to change—two, maybe three months?"

Our counselor smiles, asking, "How old are you?"

Ray answers, "Thirty-nine."

He says, "So you think I can change in a few months what took thirty-nine years to create?" Ray smiles sheepishly.

Then he says, "Jo, I think your need for everything to go smoothly makes you unable to tolerate Ray's slowness to forgive. So you take a walk, a bath, or can't lie in bed when he's angry. You hide from difficulties and withdraw."

I argue, "But I confront him."

He says softly, "But you can't stand the deafening silence."

I nod knowingly. Later, it's obvious Ray was touched; he makes passionate love to me tonight.

In the morning after the girls leave I sit on the couch and journal:

Oh my Abba Daddy, TU for life. I praise you. You are my Rock, Redeemer, Savior, and Lord. Knower of *all* things—past, present, future. You love me tenderly and want me freed. Heal me.

I remember Mom went to work when we moved to Colorado. I was seven and responsible for Rhonda when we weren't with a babysitter. I learned to cook dinners.

Dad was a perfectionist. Do I only remember the good? He read *Playboy*.

God, I'm wondering if the hold-up on the testimony for the cassette is because of what's coming to light. I had so much trouble saying "I had a happy childhood."

I felt ugly in Junior High ...

Why did I shiver when guys made out with me and I feared they'd go too far, as if *I had no control?* I remember a guy in the band unzipping my pants, then stopping as I shivered. And when I was camping, this pre-med student and I were in the trees kissing when he reached for my jeans zipper. I shook so hard he said, "You must've *really* been hurt. Don't worry, I'll stop." I cried.

Did something awful happen to me? I can't believe it was Daddy—*was it?* My mind keeps thinking a possibility but denying it.

My mind's eye flits around me now. I can't and don't want to let it settle. I must be producing this, as Mom used to say about our aches and pains.

God, I'm afraid for you to unlock the secret door of pain to the past. I think it has to do with Daddy. I'm terrified. I sit here rocking, crying, like I've done after Ray and I argue.

I'm asking myself this irrational question—did my daddy sexually abuse me? My pen feels like a cruel instrument as I write. My heart beats fast. I quiver as if chilled or sick. Daddy and I were close. He'd buy me things for my sketching. My back is tense. I—I

Abba, Daddy, my God. I think I was a victim of ...

I call Ray at work, sobbing. I can't say the word about what I've remembered. Finally he guesses. Ray's kind and grateful I shared with him. *Ray doesn't hate me. He loves me.* As I lie down I feel *again* the fondling, the sickness, the *badness.* I say the word to myself and feel God's loving arms around me. I couldn't tell myself mind over matter and write it as I remembered it. Now I pen:

God, is this why I defend myself—for protection, and to prove I'm not terrible? I was a come-on to those I dated, needing them to want me, though I couldn't go all the way because Mom said I had to be a "good girl." Did I feel I deserved a demon for a baby after seeing *Rosemary's Baby* because of *this?*

I dial our counselor and sob. I cry, "I *must* be making this up!"

He says, "Jo, it's normal to think you're lying because you don't want to believe it." I *need* to feel calm tonight when I speak.

Oh my Lord, and God, and Abba Father, I know it's *your* faithfulness I share. You'll only deepen my faith, my talk, my walk, because of this. Use me. I trust you, Lord. I've had so much joy in you, it will only increase. TU for Ray's friendship, compassion and understanding.

Tonight in L.A. I sing with more feeling than ever. At the end of my talk it *must* be the Spirit who says through me, "I've just had a memory of being sexually abused and I know God will heal this, too."

A woman about sixty in designer clothing with teary eyes whispers, "I've never told *anyone*—that happened to me, too!" I hug her tearfully, whispering back, "God *can* heal us."

You're using this to help others already, Lord!

Ray gives me a huge, warm hug, and later, embraces me again. How I need his acceptance. He says he hurt *with me* when I called. I wonder why *anyone* would love me with this in my mind.

In the morning flashes of a memory cause me to jerk in disgust and hurt as I cross my hands over my body, crying, "Don't Daddy!"

We took showers together. I weep uncontrollably, writing—"Oh God, Abba, you love me. I'm not ugly to you. I think Daddy *did* abuse me. *I feel horrible.*"

When I ask Ray if I can see our counselor he says, "Insurance may not cover it."

I cry, "I'm so upset I feel *ill. My parents are coming for a visit in two days.* I'll take out a loan!"

"You're making this an *emotional* issue. As leader of this household *I'll* make the decisions."

I yell, "Think how you'd feel if it were one of *your* girls! *I'm desperate.*"

Later we both apologize. Tears fill my eyes. "I'm sorry you thought you were marrying someone emotionally stable."

Ray wraps his arms around me. "No need for apologies. We can have a *good* marriage."

I get up and write:

"Dear Ray, Thank you so much for how you listened yesterday. If you'd reacted *any other way* it would've damaged me. I love you so much. I thank God for you because it's our relating, which we don't like, that brought me to the point of finally becoming free of what's been hidden deep inside."

In the morning Ray says I *should* get help. I see Dad's photo and cover it, then scribble:

"Though my father and mother forsake me, the Lord will receive me" (Psalm 27:10) and in my Bible column I write—"Given to me by my Abba Daddy 2/10/88 as memories sear in my soul with pain." I also remember Joshua 1:9, "Be strong and courageous ... for the Lord your God will be with you wherever you go."

As I go through journal notes with our counselor, I curl into a ball gasping with anxiety. I choke out special times with Dad that now seem ugly. I cry wrenchingly, from deep within a reservoir of pain—a grieving cry, the loss of the sweet memories.

Ray called ahead to ask the girls to be sweet and good. Melissia sings "Jesus Loves Me" and tears flow. I explain that painful memories from my childhood must be cleared up, then slip away to the bedroom to call Ruth. Her compassion and belief feel like a bear-hug from God. When Ray brings me a long-stemmed red rose, I sigh.

Lord, how amazing I know you as my loving Abba Daddy like Jesus did, and Paul wrote that we can (Romans 8:15). That I feel your acceptance. It's a miracle of grace I don't see you as an angry, abusing tyrant. It's a miracle you can use me. It's as if I had amnesia but it still affected me. Is *this* why the movie *The Color Purple* hit me so hard—because of the incest? *I wrote the word*—Incest.

As I do errands I feel afraid of *every* man. I'm a wounded finch ready for a vulture to snatch. I look at myself in the mirror and recognize me, but not me. It's as if I don't know the woman there. The hurt is so deep, pain so intense. When I spot my parents' motor home approaching, I feel dread. I don't want to touch Dad, but give him a quick hug.

While I offer them iced tea, Mom looks at me strangely, so I say, "I might act a little weird because I'm going through some stuff with a counselor."

She asks accusingly, "What kind of stuff?"

I don't answer.

I'm so glad when Ray arrives and holds me. I feel fractured. When he leaves for the store I think *I'm going to explode—I'm alone with them!*

On the patio while barbecuing I unexpectedly reveal to Mom, "I was sexually abused as a child. Memories are just now surfacing."

She cries, "Oh, *no.*"

I say through tears, "Do you believe me, Mom?"

"Of course. Why didn't you tell me?"

"I blocked it out of my consciousness as it happened. You aren't mad at me? It wasn't my fault."

"Of course not. Who was it?"

I feel trapped. "Don't ask. You don't need to know."

She says, "I was a bad parent for not protecting you. I can't imagine who we knew who came in the house and did that!" Then Mom holds me a long time while I cry.

When she asks if she can tell Dad, I answer, "If you want to."

Later I wonder *why did she assume it was in our house? It could've happened anywhere. If it were our girls I would* never *assume it was in our home.*

We take them to the coast where, Lins tells me later, Dad whispered to the girls, making them uncomfortable. I'm sad and shocked and mad. The rental movie we begin contains lewd jokes we don't expect. Dad's the only one laughing, and I feel sick.

I lurch upstairs, telling Ray when he comes up to check on me, "Say goodnight for me. I can't *stand* to be around Dad."

When I lie down the vilest of thoughts arise as I jerk this way and that.

My dad *wouldn't*—is this why a TV program made me shake violently? *God, I think the abuse happened a lot.*

I want them to leave.

Mom cries the morning they're packing up that Dad swore filthy names at her, as if he has Alzheimer's.

I say without thinking, "No, Mom, it's sin deep inside."

She responds, "I know."

We hug goodbye, but when Dad opens his door and puckers his lips like usual, I barely touch him in a hug. *No* kiss.

Ray says he wouldn't have let them come, but I couldn't get hold of them during their travels. "I think you still wanted to please your dad."

I ask Ray if I'm ugly to him. He says, "No! You're beautiful to God *and* me!"

I sob on his shoulder as he holds my hand, saying a beautiful prayer that God will heal my little girl inside. As he wraps his arms around me, I ask if he'd like to make love to me and he says, "I'd *love* to make love to you."

I'm so glad. I feared he wouldn't want me because of my ugliness.

In the morning Ruth reads me Psalm 18:18–19—"They confronted me in the day of my disaster but the Lord was my support ... he rescued me because he delighted in me."

I ask, "Why did Ken suspect Dad?"

Ruth says carefully, "Well, it's because he flirted with me. I thought he was just a dirty old man, Jo. I'm sorry to hurt you." Through tears I tell her I'm glad to know the truth.

Judie Amen's words of wisdom resound with Ray *and* me—God knew this had to come out to make me his servant, *whole,* but the enemy didn't want us together, enticing Ray to California where God worked in Ray. Then God put us together, this strong man I needed who triggered my memories and took me away from where I might not have allowed it to surface. It would be *awful* to live near my family right now. *How profound!*

As I awaken, realizing I need to live through a despicable memory, I see Ray's note—"Jo, your sweetness is beautiful to me. Love, Ray." I revel in it.

In retelling the unbelievable, feeling physical and emotional pain as if it is *now* being perpetrated on me, I wail, "He could *not* have done this!" Our counselor encourages me to reprogram myself by telling my little girl—"I have worth and value."

Why do I keep remembering fourth grade? I stayed home sick but had to do housework for Dad. He riles, "You slut!" *Am I crazy? Why would I even want to make this up? I love my family. I must trust you, God.* Tension knots my back. Bile rises in my throat and my brow furrows in pain. I did what Dad made me do—he wasn't *pleased* with me. *Oh God, help.*

I'm so grateful for God's strength to take Lindsey and Melissia to the beach for a picnic. After dinner I sit crying silent tears for little Jo who tried so hard to please Daddy with desserts. *Why, Daddy, why?*

Melissia puts her arms around me, saying, "Mommy, are you remembering your childhood again?"

I choke out, "Yes."

She whispers, "It's okay, Mommy."

During family-time she wants to write in our prayer book "Mommy would forget" but Lindsey says, "*No.* She has to remember to heal." So Melissia changes it to "Mommy would remember and heal."

One day I read and journal:

2 Corinthians 1:8—"We were under great pressure, far beyond our ability to endure, so that we despaired even of life. Indeed, in our hearts we felt the sentence of death." I *feel* that sentence—the death of my past as I had tried to paint it—wholesome and happy, thinking my father truly loved me. How could he? Verse 9—"But this happened that we might not rely on ourselves but on God." I write in the margin—"2/18/88 I claim these verses as I learn more about suffering sexual molestation." Then I pen in pronouns to personalize verses ten and eleven—*You* have delivered *me* from such a deadly peril, and *you* will deliver *me*. On *you I* have set *my* hope that *you* will continue to deliver *me* as *you* help *me* by friends' prayers. Then many will give thanks on *my* behalf for the gracious favor granted *me* in answer to the prayers of many. Without your courage, God, I want to curl up in a ball, but I have a family to care for. TU for how the

girls accepted I was sexually abused, for their hugs. I tried to explain it like their teacher would, warning them not to let others touch them.

The following day I read in Psalm 139:16—"All the days ordained for me were written in your book before one of them came to be" and I write in my Bible margin—"2/19/88 You *knew*, and were there, and loved me even as I was abused many times."

I pray, "I know you give people free choice, even for wickedness. You've proven I can trust you. I know you can work Romans 8:28 here, too. And as 2 Corinthians 1:4–5 say, you will use what I go through to help others. You *will* redeem this somehow."

While my folks are there visiting, Mom tells Rhonda, so she calls. Before guessing Dad, Rhonda suggests Grandpa, Dad's *father*. "He came on to Mom, flirting with her, so she feared being alone with him!"

Tim isn't surprised it was Dad because of the way I defended him at their house. Rhonda doesn't believe she was ever touched, but she believes me. *TU God.* I walk downstairs to see Ray holding out his arms where I feel safe.

Daily, I remind myself how faithful God is. I've claimed Psalm 40 and Ephesians 3:20 all year, since the night Ray talked about a possible move, and I now see God's incredible plan to free Ray *and* me from our painful pasts.

In a few days Ray says, "You've been such a good mom, why don't we take you out?"

Over New York pizza each of the girls say sweet things—that I'm a good mom, a good cook, they like how I sing as I tuck them in, they love me ... Ray says he orchestrated it, but they liked the idea, and he gives me a precious card thanking me for being *me*. At home Ray asks the girls to sit near him as his eyes fill with tears. He asks their forgiveness for his past anger and slapping them when they were little. Both say they never hated him.

Lindsey kisses him. "I knew it was your past and you would get over it."

"Lindsey," I remark, "it's only because your daddy *worked* on it that he got over it. Some just continue those behavior patterns."

It's such a precious time. I write a TU letter "To My Ray of Sonshine" for making it a special evening for *all* of us.

During our next session Ray explains he doesn't want to be mean, he just gets triggered by something I say or do. Tears forming, Ray says, "I don't want to go on with the anger inside. I want to love Jo more than *anything*."

Our counselor suggests I give Ray a childhood photo of me, to remind him there's a little Jo inside who needs tenderness, before he heads home from work.

Ray confesses, "We're such messes," and he says, "You've had a lot of hurt. Without permission to feel anger we bottle it up. We can't genuinely forgive until we've emotionally held people responsible—at least in our minds—for what they've done. I urge you to keep coming. You have *so* much love for each other. You'll be incredible testimonies to others when you heal. A famous pastor put counseling sessions on a credit card in order to have a good marriage with his wife."

Ray and I *heard* him say that in a sermon! He wasn't advocating going into debt, just explaining his marriage was worth *anything*, even debt for awhile.

In the morning the girls lie on top of me as I apologize for our anger affecting them. I assure them we *will* heal. Melissia gets her Bible, opening it to Psalm 147.

She reads, "How good it is to sing praises to our God ... He heals the brokenhearted and binds up their wounds ... Sing to the Lord with thanksgiving ..." (verses 1,3,7). Realizing the significance, she cries, "I just turned to it!" We all grin with joy and I kiss them as they go off to school.

Late that night I journal:

> I cried out in Ray's arms to you, God, "I *know* you allowed me to be hurt physically and emotionally because you know all things and nothing can touch me that doesn't come without your permission, like Job's experience." Ray prayed, "Your ways are not ours," and I know that's true, but *how could you watch such perversion as sexual assault?*! TU that it's okay to feel like Job and David. I can cry out, yet still know you're omniscient and you loved me even in the womb (Psalm 139:14–15).

Blackness overcomes me. I squirm. I cry, "God, *don't* let me make anything up. I have your Spirit within me. I'm *not* crazy." This time it's my white-haired deceased Grandpa.

Our counselor encourages me to see that though more memories are bubbling like hot lava to the surface of my mind, he sees a "sparkle" of self-concept growth because of how I've been *responding* to Ray instead of *reacting*. How I go to God when Ray can't help. That I haven't felt raging anger at the girls, just frustration—we three are getting along better!

The phone rings. It's Mom.

She asks, "Are you ready to tell me who and how old you were?"

I say with hurt and anger, "It was *my own father*."

Mom says flatly, "Oh. I didn't know."

"It's really been hard. You know how much I've loved Dad. Why would I make anything up?"

She says, "No, of course not."

"Mom, well, it seems there would've been *some* indication. I'm not blaming you, but I'm confused."

She states, "I didn't know *anything*."

I say gently, "Mom, I want you to know—while I spoke last week I mentioned I'd been sexually abused as a child. Just as it's helped people see God's faithfulness in other areas, they'll see his faithfulness to heal me of this, too."

She knows how my story helps others.

Mom doesn't tell me not to, but does say, "I hope you heal fast. I wouldn't want this to hurt your wonderful family."

I respond, "Mom, Ray and I have grown *closer* and sweeter these past few weeks, as well as the girls. I want you to know you were a good mom. I love you."

She says, "I love you, too."

When we're in bed, Ray prays, "Thanks for this wonderful wife who loves you more than anything and wants to be like you. Thanks for the changes you're making in me because I married her. Thanks for freeing me to love you more, and my wife. Thanks for her health. We don't take for granted how well she's doing with all this stress."

His prayer is so beautiful I can't hear the earlier tape of guilt for being honest—adding pain to Mom's life. I'm so blessed, Ray's been calling me sweetheart, baby, even beautiful. With how ugly I feel, it helps. And his teases, "frog legs," about my legs jerking up in spasms, and "rubber-band-legs," when my knees collapse, help me make light of MS.

At breakfast Melissia thanks God for each of us, then, "Thank you for putting Mommy and Daddy together so we can have a mommy again after all these years. We just praise you." *God, TU for this family. How loved I feel and how deeply I need it.*

Chapter 18

With Who I Really Am, You Still Love Me?

In a couple days I call Rhonda and Tim to see how Mom's doing.

Tim snarls, "You should *never* have told her *anything*. I've studied the Bible for years. Forgiveness is the key in Scripture, *not* confrontation!"

I feel terrible.

Tim says, "You teased her by telling her Dad has this filth in him."

I start to cry, "I told her because we're close and she knew that."

"She already feels the weight of the world with Grandmother going to a nursing home and the man she has to live with—*you of all people should know.*"

I say, "How do you think *I've* felt?"

Tim says, "Forgive. Don't dwell on it."

"I'm *not* dwelling on it, but I've got to deal with it, not stuff it."

Rhonda says, "You shouldn't go around telling everyone."

"Mom knows how God uses my vulnerability to help others. I thought she'd be glad to hear God can use this." I'm crying so hard I finally say, "I can't talk anymore. I love you," and hang up.

When I finally quit weeping, I pray for wisdom and call Mom.

I ask how she is. Mom answers, "Okay. I turn it over to God. Things that happened in my childhood are tucked away in a little corner inside. It's never affected me. It may help you, but it wouldn't help me to tell it to you. It's the past. Let it die. Go on and heal, Jo. Wash your face and put on fresh makeup and a smile, do you hear me?"

I say, "I didn't want to make you miserable. I wish you hadn't visited and found out and told Rhonda."

She responds, "God's in control of this, too."

"The only reason I would confront Dad is to give him a chance to repent."

She says, "He doesn't know what he says—"

I cut her off, "I said that two years ago and Tim bit my head off. He said, 'No way. Dad knows what he's saying!'"

"You're right, but you need to go on."

"Mom, I didn't go down the tube after Ron and you don't know the half of it. I *will* work this through."

We say good-bye and I write:

Is her denial why I never felt I could tell her? I wouldn't be believed? TU for Ray and the girls since my own family might turn against me. Tim *is* wrong, isn't he, Lord? The Bible says to confront sin in Matthew 18:15–17. In Ephesians 5:11–14 Paul says—"Have nothing to do with the fruitless deeds of darkness, but rather expose them. For it is shameful even to mention what the disobedient do in secret. But everything exposed by the light becomes visible, for it is light that makes everything visible." And Paul told believers in 1 Corinthians 5:1—"It is actually reported that there is sexual immorality among you, and of a kind that does not occur even among pagans: A man has his father's wife." *Incest.* He tells them to use tough love in verse 5—" ... hand this man over to Satan, so that the sinful nature may be destroyed and his spirit saved on the day of the Lord." Yes, Scripture teaches forgiveness, and I *want* to forgive more than anything, but confrontation is first. Search me, O God—you *know* my heart. I listen and hear, "*Jo, I love you. You are my child.*" I feel you rocking me as a baby and I'm loved by you, Abba, but I fear I can't trust myself.

"I've given you a sound mind." I sense, *"The truth must be known because you were wronged with deep hurts. I love you, Child. Rest in me."*

The company owns a condo in Palm Desert, so we excitedly drive there for a weekend of fun. Just as we begin to trek down the path at a desert museum I sigh, telling Ray, "I feel like a limp noodle." Disappointment saps what little energy the sun's blazing rays haven't used up. "I need to go inside the gift shop. You three go on."

Lindsey asks with concern, "What's wrong?"

"I'm too weak to walk around in this heat."

Hot tears sting my eyes as Melissia says, "Don't feel bad, Mommy. Have I ever told you I'm *glad* to have a mom who has MS? I'm learning so much."

She reads my thoughts as if they're emblazoned across my forehead— I'm sad MS is affecting our day, and she wants to comfort me. *How precious, Lord.*

We ooh and aah as we take the tram up San Jacinto Peak through four ecosystems. Then we scream during the roller-coaster-like-descent. After playing "Marco Polo" in the pool the girls are lounging all over Ray. It's a delightful sight, but because Ray's been avoiding me, anxiety builds. Clawing at my throat. Panic seizes me. *I don't belong here or anywhere except with you, Lord!* I run to the master bathroom and pray and sing. My racing heart slows beat by beat until I pray, "TU, Lord, for rescuing me from these thoughts. Change me." Then I write Ray a letter about my feelings.

We arrive home to a message from Mom, "Where *are* you?" so controlling I cringe.

Though we're obviously growing our counselor says, "You have a sweet personality, Jo. You just need to get stronger and tougher. What you've remembered puts women in the *hospital.* Your faith is strong, but you need Ray to be loving and nurturing, not harsh. You need to practice your letter—retreat when Ray is unsafe—don't risk being victimized. We—you, Ray, and I—need to make sure the same pattern of emotional abuse *isn't* perpetuated."

Then he prays, "God, we pray for Ray to be healed by learning to love and nurture Jo. Even at this very moment Ray would sense he needs to be sensitive to Jo."

I drive from there to a store nearby for Lindsey's birthday card and Ray rounds the corner in the aisle! He says, "Hi good-lookin'," as he kisses and hugs me. "You look *great.*"

I journal later—"You are *so* good, Lord. I feel so ugly inside-out and Ray tells me the opposite."

As I tuck Melissia in, we hold each other tightly.

She says, "I'll miss you *so* much when I'm in Colorado."

I sniffle, "Me, too, but I want you to have *wonderful* time and make lots of great memories. I'll be here when you come back! You're *not* getting rid of me."

"I don't want to," and we hug again.

It's Easter. I've already complimented the girls' mom on the beautiful dresses she sewed and we're all having a wonderful time. Ray and I have been snuggling for a few minutes in bed to begin each day. We're noticing more and more sweetness and less and less of his withdrawals and we're overjoyed as we talk about it.

Melissia comes to me after talking with her mom, saying, "I feel like crying but I don't know why."

I hold her on my lap as she says, "I miss Mommy." She begins wailing as I rock her to and fro.

In bed she cries wrenching sobs, and as Ray holds her, he cries *with her.* He's overwhelmed to *feel* her hurt instead of telling her to *quit* crying. He prays with each daughter that God will heal the hurt they have from their mother leaving them. I kneel by the bed and pray for all of them, including the girls' mom.

Ray says later, "I see increasingly why you're the best wife I could ever have." I smile, with tears of gratitude trickling from my eyes as he prays, "Thank you, God, for my wife I'm so proud of. My greatest claim in life is I'm married to her. Thank you for your wisdom in putting us together and for how sweet my love has been for her lately and how I know this will be a better relationship than I could imagine!"

More memories boil to the surface. When I realize I'm irrationally angry or can't take Ray's silence, I cry out to God for wisdom, and too often I whimper, choke, then sob out a new or fuller version of an old memory in my journal. I always ask God to keep me from making anything up. It's April and I feel I should write Dad. Mom says she knows I want to give him an opportunity to repent and hopefully change because of love:

"Dear Dad, I've told you many times, in person and letters, how grateful I was for the father you've been. I've meant every word. But four days prior to your visit I had the first of many vivid, physically painful recollections of you, as well as Grandpa, sexually abusing me. I just couldn't cope so I blocked it all out. I bore the guilt because I couldn't understand how two men I loved so much would treat me so badly—why did you do it? I feared writing because your health isn't good. You might not remember, but you also might not want to admit this. I grew up feeling unworthy, guilty, ugly, insecure, and fearful of abandonment *because* of this. I'm not writing to be mean. I'm writing to tell you I *know*. I *am* angry. I'm *so hurt* I cry from the depths of my soul, *but I will forgive you, and I love you.* More than any of the above reasons, I'm writing because I want *you* to be free from guilt and happier than ever before by asking God's forgiveness, mine, and Mom's. Oh Daddy, please do this for *yourself* so you'll have peace with God—he *will* forgive, and *I* will. Jo"

Dad calls as soon as he receives my letter, saying, "I don't remember anything but I'm sorry it caused you so much trouble."

"You're forgiven, Daddy. I love you."

He says, "So, you told Ray, huh? That's why he treated me differently. Why'd you have to tell Rhonda? Don't tell everyone. I won't live this down."

"Mom needed to know. People can't heal with things hidden. I love you."

But a counselor friend thinks I've forgiven Dad prematurely. That would be my way—make it all okay ASAP. I've just read that true forgiveness takes time for severe trauma, or it will be incomplete.[21] Our own counselor encourages me to read my journaled feelings, while suggesting Ray hold me. I begin timidly, then anger overtakes my voice as if it's finally been given permission.

After I'm spent Ray says sweetly, "I *felt* pain with you. I wish I'd been there to protect you. I love you. You're beautiful inside and out."

In the El Torito Grill this evening, Ray and I savor chili rellenos as we gaze into each other's eyes.

Ray says, "You look *really* nice."

He scoots over next to me, saying, "I want the privilege of bonding with you by helping you with the memories. I'd rather try and fail than not try. I think I'll have the courage."

I cry, "Baby, that means *so much to me.*"

I kiss him and he says, "I'm so glad you're in my life. I'd become worse and worse, filling the void with anything."

This is confirmation that as Ray supports me he'll heal! As we discuss Ray's recent offer to remain in California we agree it seems best.

Tonight, Lins cries with confusion, looking forward to being with her mom. "She says nice things, but you and Daddy tell us we're a *blessing* and a *privilege* to raise. You listen to my feelings—who will listen to my hurts this summer? And you sing to us at night."

"Oh, Lins, I'm so glad you share your feelings with me. And sometimes when I sing I'm so tired, but I feel better because I do it!"

She goes on, "And I'll miss praying with you. But I miss her and someday I might like to live with her—I wouldn't want to make you and Daddy sad."

"We want you happy. You love your mommy and she does you. A lot."

Melissia is confused, too, having nightmares, sleeping with me when Ray's gone. *God, divorce is so hard on children. I wish it never happened to them.*

On my first Mother's Day I'm given a mug saying, "I Love You Mom." Mel gives me a booklet she wrote about me saying, among other things—"The thing I do that is special to my mom is hold her when she feels bad." Tears fill my eyes. Lins hands me a card "The Recipe for Mom," saying, "You're just like that card." Ray's card says "To the Joy of My Life," then we argue, yelling like before, until we're crying in each other's arms, pleading with God to *change us.* Later I make a quick call to Mom to wish her a happy Mother's Day.

Mel prays with thanks for, "Mommy and Daddy who help me to know what's the right thing to do. It's just so funny Lord that we can sit here and talk to you as if you're right here. And you are!"

I've just recorded the song begun on the coastal steamer off Norway, so I sing it to the girls at bedtime with lots of animation as they giggle.

"My Heart Wants to Cry Out, Lord!"

Lord, I lift my eyes up to the hills, to the tall peaks surrounding my frame.
I feel so small, yet I feel so big, because you loved me so much, Jesus came.
The great power in your broad and mighty seas causes me to wonder at all your design
How you created each thing in its form and in its place,
And your love for me transcends all time.
I will never be alone without you
You always know my every hope and fear
The blessings of the life you've given through happiness and pain,
Are more than my voice can proclaim.
The clean crisp mountain air and breeze, the snowflakes flutter by so softly
The sound of chirping squirrels and birds, the pine trees with new growth so lofty
My heart wants to cry out, Lord!
I will never be alone ...

The brook bubbles through the cold thick ice. And deer walk softly on dried grass.
The enormous silence of the mountains, till clouds break in thunder, sounding a crash!
My heart wants to cry out Lord!
I will never be alone ... 22

As much as we're growing, some of the same cycle continues—Ray retreats in silence with his own termites eating away at our household of faith while I'm trying to exterminate my own.

> Give me your joy in spite of his silence. I hear, *"Don't lose hope. Your pain will bring forth gold* (I Peter 6–7). *Depend on me, not Ray, Child."* I try to lie next to my husband who can still be so intense and harsh, who says, "I can't forgive easily because of my childhood." Sometimes I fear he won't change, but there's no fear in your love. I praise you in the *midst* of this. Make our marriage holy ground for *you* to use. If I'm not careful I act defensively with my "I'll just depend on God" erecting my own barrier. We've made it past the pain before. We will again, and soar.

Ray thinks God isn't ready to free us all at once, laughing, saying we haven't hurt enough yet. "I think if we try to get out of this pain it'll be wrong. God is doing something." Then Judie Amen writes—"I know things are not easy for you, but oh, what God is doing *in you!* I stand in awe."

It's painful to say goodbye to the girls for the summer, but Ray takes me to a hotel for the weekend, running the sound equipment during my speaking engagement the following day.

He says, "I'm *so* proud of you," after watching faces respond.

A week later Ray's talking about his dad, when suddenly he cries, "He didn't show *any* appreciation for me raising five siblings by myself. He beat me instead."

Anger spikes his voice.

I'm holding him as he says, "I'm sorry, Jo, I don't want to hurt you."

"I know."

Now I squirm. My stomach churns. Pain rips through my body as I remember more. I weep uncontrollably.

Ray holds me, saying, "You're clean, baby. I'll protect you. I won't let them hurt you anymore. I love you."

I say, "Your love is sweeter than I ever imagined. Your compassion and understanding and caring overwhelm me, but I'm so scared sometimes. I need you to love and hold me."

"Jo," our counselor says, "God, in his grace, didn't allow the memories until you had a man you could trust to help you through it."

He prays for my emotional healing as well as physical healing of MS while Ray holds me tightly as I sob.

Ray leans inside my car as I continue weeping, saying, "You're beautiful. You mean the world to me. I'd use every penny I have to get you help to heal. I really *felt* your pain. I hurt *with* you and I was angry at them. I *will* protect you, sweets."

At home I curl up beside him and he holds me for hours as we watch an old movie. Then he makes love to me and I sob from a place so deep inside I can't locate it.

I whisper, "All I ever wanted was to be was cherished. I feel so loved."

Mom calls *while* I'm reliving more of the memory. *Help me, God.* She wants to know how I *really* am so I answer, "I'm reliving the *worst* memory of all."

She says, "Oh no." I say with hurt, "I can't understand how you couldn't have known *anything*, Mom. Unless I hid it so well, maybe because of threats."

She says soundly, "I did not know a thing."

I tell Mom I love her, then curl into a ball like a roly-poly bug to protect myself, feeling terrible for hurting her. Ray reaches out his arms to hold me while praying my family won't turn on me, but if they do his love will be enough.

Capping off a seafood anniversary dinner overlooking the ocean, I read what Ray wrote in his card—"You are so very dear to me. Thank you for showing me what love is and helping to teach me. Love, Ray." Then I sing the song I wrote, his eyes tearing up:

"First Year"

It's funny how we look at life, thinking all seems clear
God would use me tenderly to help my husband heal.
At times the days were full of fun, but fears inside me grew
Trusting in agape love was all that we could do.
And I dreamed of being cherished, of knowing I was loved
Wanting smoothness and commitment, and help from God above.
Then the memories surfaced; the pain was so severe.
I feared I must be crazy and you might not endure.
But your love comes sweetly to me, so gently holding tight.
Our sharing tears o'rwhelms me; our hearts seem to take flight.
Oh I dreamed of being cherished, of knowing I was loved
Not guessing that in God's design my pain makes your love shine.
With such joy I know I'm cherished, the depth of bonding grows.
And our great Lord's faithfulness is proved as our first year draws to a close.

Following my assessment two days later our counselor says, "Ray, your character *has* changed as you've allowed yourself to be vulnerable."

Then I get home and read Mom's card—"When the going gets tough, the tough get ice cream! Love, Mom." *Her buck-up-get-over-it!* She writes she would never have allowed anything to happen to me by Dad or Grandpa. She didn't notice anything going on—*do not blame me!*

Oh Abba, where was she all those times I was abused? Make me a better mom because of the healing of memories. *Don't let me discount the girls.* I need a forgiving heart. I feel guilt creeping up on me like a spider, telling me I've done wrong in confronting sin. Luke 17:4 says—"If your brother sins, rebuke him and if he repents forgive him." In that order. Lord, I just want to be in your will. Touch others through me for your glory.

When Ray comes home from work he asks, "Baby, what do you want from your mom?"

I sob as I say, "I want her to say, 'I'm sorry I wasn't there for you. I'm sorry I didn't protect you' and nothing else. No excuses or reasons."

Ray rocks me as I continue sobbing. We decide I should write Mom a letter, which Ray approves. I tell her I'm hurt and angry. That I'm not blaming her but I just needed to tell her how I felt. "All I really want to hear from you is … Healthy people happen because of dealing with emotions—not cover-up and 'stuffing.' I desire wholeness for all of us. I love you."

I journal—"I think Mom can't admit she *wasn't* there for me."

In a few days Ray and I call and Ray explains what I need from her.

Mom cries, "I'm finally at the point I can tell myself I've been a good mother." Ray affirms that by telling what he sees in me, but by the end of the call he sees she hasn't met my need for compassion.

We're telling our counselor about the conversation with Mom and he notices Ray's gentle affection. He says, "Ray, I haven't seen such a dramatic change in *anyone* in a *long* time. You two have such a ministry. Someday I hope you'll write your story for others. Jo, remember you *are* walking with the Lord."

When Ray sees the insurance statement, he says tearfully, "That's the best spent money ever, and I couldn't see it! I'm *such* a bonehead at times."

I don't say a word, but inside I'm smiling.

Our neighbor, Linda, is moving, and I feel happy and sad. She tells us we were a big influence orchestrated by God to change her life, turning her to Jesus.

All I can say is, "What a privilege it was! I'll *really miss* you." *Abba, place us in a neighborhood where we can again be used to draw others to you.* We're looking to buy rather than rent.

Ray and I have been in training for the MS150 Bike Tour to raise funds for MS. The ride takes off from the San Diego train station with a 100-mile route over two days passing through beautiful country. After camping overnight we decide next year we'll opt for a hotel room. We didn't get enough sleep with our sore muscles on the ground. Though we arrive at the finish next to last, who cares? *We made it.* What an exhausted week for me afterwards. I experience so much MS nerve fiber pain in my spine Ray tells me go ahead and cry. He holds me as tears pour, praying for me. I'm amazed.

It's delightful to see the girls again, but they struggle with "Jo" and "Mom." I discover they couldn't give me gifts they made because their mom felt so bad.

> I'll never be a *real* mom, but I can give them a love for you. It requires relinquishing the bittersweet feeling that I love them so, and would have wanted them, but their mom left them at one and three—how unfair. I must forgive her. I feel like a velveteen mom and that needs to be enough, Lord. It was precious when Lins read the *Velveteen Rabbit*[23] to Melissia and me last year. I'd never heard of it, but as the story unfolded about a stuffed bunny loved to thread-bareness, who was told earlier by the Skin Horse in the nursery that is how one becomes *real,* Lins cried, "You're a velveteen mom!"

Lins says, "I wanted to call you 'Mom' but I constantly got flak about it." Melissia also says she wants to call me "Mom." When Ray comes home he wants it settled. I take a walk so they don't feel pressured during their discussion, and they both decide to call me that and suffer the consequences. Ray says he'll back them, and he's proud they worked through their feelings.

Lins states, "If she hadn't left, she wouldn't have this problem. She knew Daddy would marry again someday."

After thanking God for her family who loves her, Mel cries deeply. She grasps me, sobbing, "I'm afraid you're going to leave me."

I assure her I *will never leave her.*

She says, "If you leave there will be a big hole in my heart. So big it will cover my whole heart!"

I smile, "I'll be here in the morning." She grins and hugs me.

Our counselor's face lights up about my cassette including my own songs and testimony as he says, "It's really good. I look forward to using it with my clients."

But I tell him I feel vulnerable having admitted I was a victim of sexual child abuse. "I feel fractured. I mourn deeply with no provocation. I'm depressed at times like never before and exhausted trying to figure out who I really am. A battle rages within me when I try to tell myself I'm God's beautiful creation. It's as if I could *not* be. Three days ago I stood looking in the mirror, cocked my head and cried as I told myself, 'You're a clean little girl.'"

Tears escape my eyes as he says, "It's all normal. Tell little Jo it's okay to feel all the feelings," so I do.

I'm dealing with scary MS symptoms as well. My eyes jump from word to word when I read if I'm fatigued, and I have trouble focusing them sometimes. Dizziness blindsides me. It's a tough time. And Lins can be *so* stubborn and willful and she questions everything and argues incessantly.

> Lord, make me a parent who does not say, "I'm proud of you but—" like I did this morning before she left for school! I assure her constantly her grades do not determine our love, then this. Lift her in spite of my words! TU for strength to tell her not to talk to me without respect yesterday. She apologized. Bless us with good times to negate the bad. Give me wisdom. I butt heads with her too often. Bring up whatever hurts cause me to become angry with her. I love them both so much. I can't imagine asking them to do what you asked of your Son, Jesus—to die for murders, rapists, gossipers, liars, people like me …

I've struggled with how *my own dad* could do what he did and seem so normal on the outside. Now I know that's how it's covered up. I realize after calling my folks to see how they're doing I grieve the loss of relationship with Mom. I also feel guilty that I'm not the doting, sweetly loving daughter I used to be—the pleaser who made everything as good as could be. It's not helping that Ray is defensive. *Is he suppressing anger about something?*

Our counselor says, "Ray, you're pulling away from feeling responsible for your mother and her fears, so you're distancing from your wife." Ray had told us how terrified he felt when his mom came to him for protection from her husband's beatings and Ray knew he'd be swept aside by his dad.

He says as I cry next to him, "I won't leave you. I want our marriage to be the best. I love you so much."

Besides speaking for luncheons and church banquets, I'm speaking for my first retreat at Arrowhead Springs, California. I pray, "Oh, Abba Daddy,

I want to be a drink offering poured out for you as a sacrifice for others to be brought to *you*. TU for allowing me this privilege." For the first time I say the word "incest," and women respond with tears and private personal sharing.

When I return home Ray gives me a mug with these words on it—"In all ways and for always I will be in love with you." *Ahhhhhhh.*

It's two days later and I'm still tired out, but I know the retreat was worth it. As I meet Ray at our counselor's, I begin saying, with anger building, "My greatest pain is my mother not being there for me!"

Ray understands feeling abandoned. His parents didn't show up for visits at the foster homes, and Ray had to make excuses to his two brothers. Six siblings were split into three different homes. We cry together as we realize God didn't give us what we wanted in a relationship, but what we *needed*— each other—a spouse who would trigger us so we could both heal.

Chapter 19

Birth Family Denies While New Family Cherishes

I can not *believe* what my mother has done—called my husband to manip-ulatively sway him to the family's side! They all believe I'm making more of this than it was. Ray said he believes *everything* because he's held me as I relived memories and *felt* the pain, fear, and shame. He told Mom he had to encourage me to confront and *not* feel guilty because I wanted to protect them. My anger dissolves into tears. *I love them so much.*

In the morning we're all scrubbing and I'm ready to drop. Ray says with cute toughness, "You lie down right now or you'll get it!"

I say, "I can't 'till I get a kiss," so he kisses me. I tease, "I can't 'till I'm tucked in."

He calls, "Girls, tuck Mommy in and *don't* let her get up and work!"

Lins says, "Daddy says you have to lie down so you have energy for a date tonight."

I respond, "You go down and tell Daddy to rest, too." She grins and runs downstairs.

Mel comes to tuck me in and lies on top of me, saying, "Daddy could've searched the whole world and not found a better little bear for himself. You're *just right* for Daddy."

They love it when Ray's protective and loving.

Then Rhonda's letter drills holes in my boat of emotions, and I sink into a sea of guilt. She twists things I've written and condemns my spirituality. She believed me at first about Dad's abuse, but when I implicated Grandpa she became suspicious, since she brought him up. She says it sounds like I grew up in another family. She's not angry, yet her letter is full of anger. She tries to disprove each instance. It's all Ray and close friends can do to hoist me out of the water in which I flounder.

I'm reminded reconciliation differs from forgiveness, which God expects, because he forgave me—and I want. I *miss* my family. I rushed to forgive Dad because I needed to fix things. It's taken me months to admit he took *no* responsibility. The goal of reconciliation requires perpetrators *accept* responsibility for pain rendered and not deny anger resulting from it, but I can forgive without reconciliation, and that will free *me* from bondage to bitterness. I begin listing Bible verses about truth:

> Know the truth and it will set you free (John 8:32). God desires truth in our inner self (Psalm 51:6). God searches for it (Psalm 44:21). I'm to examine myself (1 Corinthians 11:28). Jesus confronted the woman at the well about herself (John 4:16). And when Tamar was raped by her brother Amnon, her other brother Absalom took her in, but hated Amnon. King David, though furious, did not punish his son; he did nothing. Murder eventually ripped the family apart due to unresolved feelings (2 Samuel 13:1–29).

When Judie Rice meets me off the freeway halfway between our homes for lunch I'm warmed by her compassion. She personalizes John 15:27, "And you also, Jo, must testify. It costs. You will encounter hatred for being honest. But those God uses are those who've been hurt deeply."

I cry, praying on the way home, "It will hurt if I lose my birth family. Help me, Lord."

Now I hear Mom will not concede *anything* happened to me after preschool—I made it up from reading, television, movies. She now denies things she *agreed* to months ago! I must *face the family,* and there will be *no relationship with me* if it means conceding to my memories. *They will try to annihilate my "stories."* My chin trembles. Fresh sobs choke me. I ache as if punched in the stomach. I love them. I don't want to hurt my family.

> I love you, Abba. You loved me first and I sense your love for me because I have loved you and have believed that Jesus came from you (John 16:27). You've shown me these memories so I'll have peace. I haven't lied. In this world I will have trouble. I hear, *"Take heart, Child, Jesus has overcome the world"* (John 16:33).

At our counselor's, Ray says he's just realizing he *always* gets depressed at Christmas and holidays. Eyes filled with tears, he says he doesn't remember *anything* good, only drinking, disappointments, and more drinking. He and his siblings stayed in the car while his parents got drunk in a bar. I compassionately touch his arm. He admits he's more intense now. He wants to read the book about children of alcoholics. *PTL!*

Watching the girls sing in Christmas programs brings tears to our eyes as Ray and I hold hands. I recall our surprise 40th birthday party for Ray at Chevy's where the girls wore poodle skirts I'd sewn. Fun at Knotts Berry Farm and Disneyland with me in the wheelchair. Camping near the Mt. Palomar Observatory. Taking the girls to Souplantation after church to fill their "hollow legs." Trips to Dana Point. Camping with Melissia's Girl Scout troop.

As the girls say, "We have *fun.*"

After Christmas the pastor at a large church introduces me for my program replacing his sermon, "Sometimes you meet someone who's walked with the Lord, and he's evident in their life, and you find out it's due to pain."

A woman calls, saying they're from alcoholic homes, she's in counseling for molestation, and she thought, *great, another all-is-perfect-when-we-walk-with-the-Lord-testimony.*

"But," she says, "My husband cried throughout it! You touched our *entire* family."

I realize I've felt so much blame it's hard to think I deserve goodness; or the pastor's introduction! Yet Psalm 119:71 says—"It was good for me to be afflicted so that I might learn your decrees." This is why you're evident in me at times—because I love you, Lord, *no matter what happens.* I heard victims feel anger at *themselves* because they could be abused. I feel that, but you allowed abuse in your sovereignty, because you let sin take its own course. I've also heard healing must take place before confronting family, and this is a mistake I made. Without confrontation, though, the victim feels like the sinner who conceals a sin and will not prosper (Proverbs 28:13). Lord, heal me of all my hurts. Use this for your glory.

Today, the leader of my small group says he sensed healing when he realized he couldn't "save" his family. Wracking sobs fold my body in two as I cry, "I love you, but I can't save you from this."

I *know* I wasn't taking revenge. Later I read the effects of abandonment in abuse, realizing how easily I've felt overwhelmed, guilty, blaming myself. *I've had to work hard to give my fears to you, Lord.*

As we face our counselor, Ray says a foster mother made him read the Bible every night while saying, be strong, don't cry or feel sad about his parents. Ray tells his little boy it's okay that he felt this, then cries harder than he has since his mother died of the effects of alcoholism when he was twenty-five.

It's our first ski trip to Mammoth, California! The girls take lessons while Ray and I ski—it feels *sooooo* good. I've missed it. We're having such fun, not letting cross words affect us. When we all ski together the girls say they love it and can hardly wait to go again! I'm thrilled. Then I write:

Abba, *why* does Lins push my buttons? She's so like I was—I *am?* I need to *love* her. I spoke with such anger she ran to the kitchen and cried into her hands with fear. I apologized. I must have so much pain inside still. I must keep hoping in your power to change the blackest soul. I feel so unworthy of your love, but I know it's your grace and mercy that makes me yours, not anything I do.

A few weeks later while we're watching a movie I realize once again the fear I put into Lindsey and ask her forgiveness.

"It's okay. You were angry about your childhood."

"That's no excuse. I never want to do that again."

A new level of an old memory surfaces and I whisper, "Abba, help me remember so I can be free." Ray holds me in his arms as I cry, "I'm afraid you'll think I'm disgusting."

He says softly, "I love you, baby."

After I choke out the memory I say, "I looked in the mirror today and said, 'You're ugly.'"

He says, "You're not. You're beautiful."

Lins opens the door, lies down and rubs my back. I begin sobbing again.

Ray whispers, "God's using our love to heal you." He says to Lins, "No one let Mommy cry or said they were sorry, or 'I'll protect you.'"

Is this good for the girls? I know they're becoming sensitive to friends' problems and praying for them, but still—

Later I say, "I promise to work at seeing you as committed to me and making our marriage good—not to think of you with fear you'll be like those who've hurt me."

Ray, sincerely touched, says, "Let's write in our Bibles that commitment." I cry for joy because our counselor suggested this *a year ago*. When I brought it up before, we argued.

Ray has our Bibles on the coffee table with a pen after dinner. When he writes in mine next to the "love chapter," 1 Corinthians 13—"I will never abandon you, but keep you always 2/16/89 Ray," I begin to cry, fighting back deep sobs. We kiss and I write in his—"I will never leave you but will faithfully love and live with you till I die. I love you, Jo." Ray tears up as well.

Then Grandmother calls to ask what's between Mom and me. *God, do I tell her?*

Without specifics, I say Dad abused me and she responds, "Them telling you you're sick or crazy or lying is an easy out. I believe you and I'll pray. I know it happened to some of my students. We need to let God work now." I'm immensely grateful and relieved Grandmother believes me, and she'll pray.

Now Ruth and I get to minister together again in Colorado. My family's good-byes were loving, with Melissia's, "Eight days is *too long*, Mommy."

I'm blessed to hear one woman say, "You gave me hope it *will* quit hurting so badly," as we hug tearfully. At a church concert an acquaintance says she played my recording for five hours to get through a painful night.

I'm thoroughly enjoying my visit with the Peters' then Ruth takes me to see Mama. She wants to meet my family.

Mama says regarding the incest, "They need to face it. We love you so much. I pray every night for you."

My week is topped off like a cherry crowning a sundae by skiing with Anne, then Dave fixes us dinner. I *needed* this—I miss my friends. I do not visit my parents, and it feels like a death-sentence when we all decide it's best I don't see Grandmother.

I'm only back one day when she calls again—*angry*.

"I grew up learning to put the past behind me and not let it bother me. They did that. Your dad was young then. The devil, not God, wants you to bring this up to hurt your ministry!"

I explain my desire for our family to live in the truth like Jesus teaches. "I *love* you, Grandmother."

I hurt for her; the family is all she has. I've lost them all. My anguish prompts waves of sorrowful weeping on our bed. Soon all my family comforts me, saying I'm safe, they'll protect me.

One of the girls says, "Our love for you is as great as the whole universe."

This is precious, but is it good for the girls?

Ray says, "I fell in love with you the first night we went out, and I've been in love with you ever since. You're beautiful." He sings a song about always being there for me whether I'm lost or falling apart, and I cry. Ray says, "I'm happier than I've *ever* been in my life," as he kisses me.

I sniffle, "When you care for me I feel like a rose covered with dew, the morning sun shines on me and I glisten and smell fragrant."

Then we discuss the girls and I journal:

Help me think *before* I use a sharp tone—like with Mel yesterday, forcing me to apologize. Stop me from jumping to conclusions without asking questions and keep me from interrupting their answers. TU for the joy of parenting. *Every* time Ray leaves town they test to see if I'll reject them, especially Melissia. We can have silly moments and sweetness, then she rejects *me*. I tell her I *won't* leave. They also have more aches and pains and I'm responding like Mom, uncompassionate! You're allowing this so I will change. You're repairing the weaknesses in *me* (I Peter 5:10).

But Ray reminds me the girls are masters at manipulation, especially with me. Even so, Lins' teacher says she talks incessantly about Ray and me. She's so happy it's almost as if she's afraid it will end.

When I ask her about that Lins says, "No, I'm just *proud* of you," and we hug.

Now I need to ask Melissia's forgiveness for swatting her behind. *She apologized for her attitude, Lord, but I should never do that in anger. TU for patiently teaching and forgiving me, but change me. I don't ever want to swat them!* Ray and I explain that we love her, though she needs discipline.

She says, "You're very special parents! And you thought you'd never get married because of your MS!"

When Melissia shares how Ray and my arguments force her into their shower with her radio as she curls up, crying, I say, "I'm *so* sorry. It's both our fault, but it's less and less," and she agrees. *God, how awful. We've got to change quickly!*

Grandmother calls for the third time, saying, "Forget this and drop it! Act like a Christian. We want to bring you back into our family like it used to be!"

I sigh, "That's not up to me."

She snaps, "*You* did this to us!" and I wince.

"I haven't done anything but bring up the truth, so we can *all* heal. I love you, but I need you to stop saying these things."

My eyes brim with tears until the mail arrives with Mom's letter. She writes I haven't been cut off if that's what I think, and if I expect more than a newsy letter, I'd better toss it! *Crazy-making par excellence after saying last fall we wouldn't have a relationship unless I recant.*

Then I hear from my former counselor in Colorado who thanks me for my essay. Diane *did* question in her mind if my family could've been as good or encouraging as I portrayed them. She affirms how bizarre it feels—this stuff *does* happen in families.

She passed around copies to the counseling staff, saying, "This woman knows who she is in Christ and *still* couldn't have victory until she dealt with victimization."

I feel validated just when I crave it. I've battled so much guilt over the letters of confrontation.

I jot on my birthday:

TU that I didn't kill myself, become a whore, or slave to drugs or alcohol. TU the best is yet to come as I love you and let you shine through me, bringing you praise and glory. TU for showing me how to nourish little Jo last night as I cried "It's okay to live now. It's okay to be confused about Mommy and Daddy. To love them and hate what they're doing. To want their nourishment yet want to say I let go of you." TU I could separate *Grandmother's* conviction from yours, Lord. When she told me to listen to you, I told her I *am*. TU for my wonderful family.

We're at a restaurant in Dana Point harbor and I entrust Lindsey with the sound equipment as Mel helps. Lins handles it beautifully, but just when I'm telling the audience how to know Jesus loves them, a boat's radio interferes—with conversation leaking through my Bose speakers! I joke about it, then explain again.

Mel prays at dinner, "Thank you for my mother and what she does and how *four* people became Christians even though the devil tried to prevent them from hearing! Help them grow."

God, you're so creative!

Today the girls are crabby, but Mel sits crying, and I ask her why.

She says, "I don't want to be here. I don't belong. I don't know why I'm alive," as tears roll down her cheeks.

I pull her into my arms and say, "I'm not leaving you. You're *so* special and important to me. Daddy, Lins and I love you. Life wouldn't be the same without you. Go ahead and cry."

Mel cries from deep within, moaning, "Help me."

I hold her tightly. "I'm here. I love you, Melissia."

I cry with her and she eventually falls asleep.

Three hours later she wakes, saying, "Thank you for helping me awhile ago, Mommy."

I respond, "I was glad to. I'm *never* leaving."

I answer the phone later to hear about Ruth's conversation with Mom, since she and Ken will retrieve things stored at my folks'.

Mom cried, "I wanted Jo to have to come get her things so she'd talk to us."

Ruth said, "Jo doesn't feel there can be any reconciliation without acceptance of the abuse and some compassion."

Mom said, "I disagree. Jo should consider this as something that happened and *go on!*" Mom told Ruth she admits to some of it, but not all.

Ruth said, "There is *no* reason for Jo to make any of this up. *I believe her.*"

I say, "Thanks for backing me, Ruth," shaking my head sadly.

Before we head for Colorado we celebrate our second anniversary. The Bronco's stuffed with clothing and we four as we drive to Ouray to take the girls jeeping. Black Bear is number 5 out of 5 difficulty, ending up in Telluride, and Ray slides cautiously on shale.

One of the girls says, "Well, if we fall off the mountain, at least we'll all go to heaven!" and we laugh nervously. I'm having a thrill of my life—I *love* this road.

As Ray and I stay with Ruth and Ken, they listen compassionately, then we pick the girls up from their mom's to take them to Anne and Dave's, and we visit Mama and Papa, who are delighted to meet my family.

After our drive home hauling a full trailer, Ray and I struggle.

Our counselor says, "Ray, your wife is a little afraid of you."

I cry, "A *little*? A *lot*," with tears running down my face.

Ray strokes my hand, "Jo's fears trigger my anger. *Every* time my mom was irrational I wanted to yell, 'Get it together, you're my mom! I need you to be in control of yourself!'"

Tears overflow Ray's eyes. I hold him as he says, "I'm sorry. I don't mean to make you afraid."

I whisper, "I know. I'm trying to see the little boy who's hurting."

God uses concerts in Laguna Niguel and San Jose to *prove* I'm doing his will in telling about the incest, because afterwards women tearfully reveal their own secrets. After my second concert, Ray and I make wonderful memories in San Francisco. We're overcome with happiness to make it *five days* without conflict!

The summer speeds by. We pick the girls up at the airport, surprised to see their faces heavily made up. Ray says, "Their mom will encourage things we wouldn't because she wants their acceptance. We may have problems every time they go to her."

Soon after their return Melissia sits on my lap with tears filling her eyes as she says for the first time, "I'm mad she left me."

"It's okay to be angry."

Mel bawls, "I want my mommy."

I comfort her, then Ray holds her as I pray silently, *God, heal all of our hurts.*

When Ruth recounts her recent talk with Mom, I hear again I must *face the family.* It's up to *me.* Mom said I blame her for everything. Thankfully, I sent copies of all the letters I'd written to Ruth so she could honestly say, "I've read the letters Jo wrote. I didn't read that. I saw nothing but truth, love, even tenderness."

She tells me, "Jo, she sounds hard and bitter. Your letters said nothing to cause them to react as they have, except guilt to be covered up. I fear she'll take it to the grave, and even though you forgive in your heart, it may not mean reconciliation. Christ offered forgiveness to many who haven't received it and been reconciled to him."

I must remember this and what a counselor friend said, "Your motive was pure in writing the letters. If only we'd known what was ahead."

Though Ray and I are learning to diffuse our frustration before it becomes an argument, I'm thrilled he's attending an Adult Child of Alcoholics group at church. Afterwards, he brings home a huge bouquet of flowers with a sexy card, looking like an embarrassed schoolboy infatuated with love as I read it, hug and kiss him. The girls spied him through the window and ran out of their room to watch my face. At dinner we explain what triggered our argument yesterday, how we handled it wrong and what *would've* been best. Ray says, "Couples will argue, but there is a right and a wrong way."

My study group is helping me realize I don't need to feel guilty, but rather just ask for help without defensiveness. *And,* I need to be aware of subtle need to "control" things—like *I* want them to happen. I journal— "TU for tough times of being triggered, because when I realize *why,* I can heal further, and *that's* when I've learned to soar!"

The following week I have the awesome opportunity to share my story and sing before a large, expressive group. The next day I'm bushed. I can't even bring in grocery bags on my luggage carrier. A neighbor happens by like an angel. I collapse on a chair and cry in gratitude that God answered my prayer for help. *Does this mean I'm not trusting you for strength, Lord, or just putting myself on a guilt-trip again?* I'm thinking *this is what Joni would call one of those I-wish-I-had-use-of-my-hands-days,* when the phone rings and I'm shocked to hear Joni Eareckson Tada ask how I am! A friend of hers heard me speak yesterday and Joni wanted to call. I tell her how she's touched my life so often. How her marriage to Ken gave me courage to risk again. I can't stop smiling.

Though I have retreats ahead, one day I realize my ministry isn't what it used to be, but must come second to my family anyway. Then I push the recorder to find a message from the Joy Program on TBN asking me to sing in a couple months! *TU, Lord!*

Next Sunday we return from a fun *and* frustrating long family weekend in Palm Desert to a message, "Jo, it's your mother. Call me back when you get a chance." The voice is hard, like cement in a brick wall. Ray's shocked, but I'd *sensed* she called. I ignore it to see our counselor about my latest, *new*, disgusting memory. What I wrote in my first letter was the *tip* of the iceberg.

When we return Mom's call, Ray sits holding one phone across from me at the kitchen table (with Mom knowing) as I grasp the other.

She touts, "I hope you never make any mistakes as a mother."

I respond, "I do, daily, but I ask forgiveness."

She says, "I didn't think I did anything to ask forgiveness for!"

When Ray mouths *tell her what you've recently remembered and how you felt abandoned,* I do.

She says, "Come off it, Jo! I didn't know anything. I was at work."

Ray and I shake our heads.

I say, "This is getting us nowhere, Mother."

"You're right. It isn't. I hope you're feeling okay, Jo. I love you very much."

I tell her how I'm doing and that I pray for her to heal, then cry all evening. *Interesting—she said she was at work so she didn't know about the incest. Recently she would not accept anything after preschool, yet she didn't begin working until I was seven.*

The day before I'm on the Joy Program I'm assaulted with guilt.

I feel *bad*—should never have written—I'm lying—deranged. I'm naked on TV for all to see, singing off-key—pride. I put on the armor of God to stand against the enemy's lies. He wants me paralyzed by fear. I *will not* be! I have your power. I can't do it, but *you* can! I've been afraid to trust that *I* can get out of the way and let you do it through me. It's like I don't deserve to have you work through this filthy vessel. But this child isn't to blame—little Jo was a victim! You died for *me*. I pray out of your glorious riches, Abba and Lord, you strengthen me with your power through your Spirit, so that Christ may dwell in my heart through faith (Ephesians 3:16–17).

As Ray and I wait in the studio, in walks an author to talk about his book. We tell him how it touched us.

He says, "Ray, you have a sweet spirit."

I touch Ray's arm, saying, "He does."

After I sit on a stool and sing, the interviewer sits down beside me, casually beginning a short question and answer period. Then he and the author talk, who brings *me* up as an example of someone who has every reason to be angry, thinking life is unfair, but he doesn't sense any bitterness in me because of working through my past.

I know I've been working through the anger healthily and am healing and forgiving them.

We're excited I've been asked to sing and share again. I find out after the live taping that Roene prayed all day, interceding in the gap. *TU, Lord!*

After dinner, which Ray buys for his worn-out-though-flying-in-the-clouds-wife, Melissia sings her own ditty, "How much is that mommy in the window? She's not for sa-le, she's mine!"

Lindsey pipes up, "Have you noticed how immature and silly boys are? Have you noticed how Daddy still acts that way sometimes?" and we all cackle.

As I get ready for bed after finding it impossible to read because my eyes bounced from word-to-word, I realize again I must be careful—with every heightened symptom I risk a more serious MS attack.

On Thanksgiving eve I leave a message on my parents' recorder—"I'm thankful for all of you. I'm even thankful for the painful things I've remembered because God works it all together for good. I love you all. Have a happy Thanksgiving."

In December, after I sing two songs the interviewer tells me he'd like to have me back for a total show of my testimony. "How 'bout your husband, too?"

Ray agrees, saying, "I couldn't have accepted this part of your ministry a year ago—including me in it. God is in this happening *now.*"

As I prepare in prayer, next to Psalm 119:74—"May those who fear you rejoice when they see me, for I have put my hope in your word," I write—"Help others through our story." During the show I tell bits of my past in answer to the interviewer's questions, then he asks Ray how he felt as I sobbed over the phone about my first memory.

Ray tilts his head thoughtfully. "Well, you know, it scared me. I came from a very abusive background with lots of hurts. I was emotionally closed, afraid I would need to be a feeling person. But I had learned about sharing my feelings from several good books. I'd read what God says in the Bible about what it means to love my wife. I believed God's promises were true and wanted to test them. I committed to stick with my wife through therapy, sitting right beside her, so I could bond with her. I just sensed that God wanted to bless me through experiencing my wife's pain."

Then the interviewer asks Ray what he would like to tell men who want to run the other way from their wives' hurts.

Ray's voice grows more passionate as he answers, "I would urge any man who desires a super, loving relationship with his wife to be there for her. Reach out. Put your arms around her and hold her when she needs to cry. Show her the compassion that Jesus Christ showed the Church. That pleases God so much, he'll bless you. It doesn't happen overnight, and we've had struggles, but the joys we've experienced have been great."

As Ray squeezes my hand, he's asked if my past brought up his hurts. Did he have to deal with his own?

Ray smiles and says, "That's the beauty of God putting us together. He wanted my wife's need for compassion to help *me* become whole. As God gives me strength and courage to show her acceptance and love, I vulnerably deal with my own reasons for being afraid—the hurts from my past. Through that God is showing me *I* am accepted and loved by not only my wife, but him as well! He's shown me if I'm faithful to work at being vulnerable in our relationship—and it is a lot of work—he'll bring healing, give me joy, and help me love my family. It's a process."

There isn't a dry eye in the filming crew as we finish.

Chapter 20

Birth Mother Woes as Healing Continues, MS Worsens

On Christmas morning we hold hands while we watch the Joy interview. After opening gifts a sales rep in Dallas calls, says he surfed channels, recognized us, and watched it all!

Judie Amen says she could see a prophecy being fulfilled—that Ray would someday share as well. She sees how impacting it is with the love and acceptance in our faces. When I tell Ray, he smiles broadly.

Then a distraught man who looked us up through information after seeing the program asks Ray how he can help his wife. After encouraging him, Ray says, "I don't think I'm ready for lots of these calls."

I realize as I'm answering a stack of mail I *too* feel overwhelmed—I'm still remembering *new* horror. Just today I thought about the special day in seventh grade when Daddy picked me up at the bus-stop during a blizzard. His charming smile elicited my own. The happy, bonding memory turns into another instance of filthy name-calling, degrading sex, threats to keep quiet, and shame so toxic I can barely journal through nauseous wailing, wearing me onionskin thin.

Now Lins is sick, saying I don't believe she feels bad. I ask God *search my heart,* and realize I don't feel I can be honest about MS symptoms or fatigue, so I'm projecting that onto Lins! I explain how I feel, apologize, and comfort her lovingly.

I must give myself permission to have crash days. I'm too worn out to love well.

As we sit in our session, tears pour down my face while I say, "I've had so much nerve fiber pain since Christmas, and a natural fear about MS, I'm thinking, *What if I get worse—will you stay with me? Will your eyes wander because I cease being attractive to you?* Healthy denial is one thing, but I have been worse lately."

Ray's eyes fill with tears. "I married you for your mind and your kindness and your integrity, not how you look, though I *do* enjoy your body and looks. I'm not ashamed of you—I'm *proud.* I don't care if you need to use a wheelchair, or even if you're in bed. The you I married is *inside* your body."

I'm crying as Ray says, "I love you. I'll never leave you."

"I'll never leave you either. I'm afraid to tell how bad I feel sometimes because of my upbringing."

Suddenly I cry mournfully, "Don't leave me alone sick with Daddy, *please* Mommy."

Ray holds me while emotions from an old memory rip through me in sobs, whispering, "I won't leave you."

When I finally calm down Ray says, "Jo's been wonderful. She's taught me compassion. She's a gift."

Then Ray returns to work and I home to Melissia, who cries, "I want my mommy."

I hold out my arms and she wails, "She's mine, why can't I have her?"

I answer, "It's not fair. It's not your fault. It's okay to cry. You're precious—so special and unique. I love you *so* much. You're the greatest little gift I've been given."

She cries for a while, and when Ray comes home, he asks me how I feel.

"I hurt at first, but reminded myself I'm not Melissia's natural mother. By God's grace I'm a caretaker."

I'm a velveteen mom earning her right. I pray, "Keep reminding me I'm here to meet *their* needs, not them to meet mine."

After dealing with Lins, I cry, "Lord, keep pointing out my sin. My behavior is *so* immature! I felt responsible for Lins' feeling overwhelmed by two chores along with homework, so I discounted her with 'Come off it!' just like *I* heard. I apologized. I *don't* want to be like this."

We've skied in the mountains nearby, but after we go to Mammoth I journal:

> TU for saving me from hypothermia! I knew something was wrong when I felt like napping on the slope—then I crumpled in a heap, my muscles hard as iron. I lay against Ray covered by coats as I shivered uncontrollably. I kept praying silently, "In my weakness you are strong, Lord." The ski patrol skied me to their emergency unit on a sled. I prayed, "Keep me alive, Lord. *I want to live!*" My body convulsed with spasms. I couldn't open my eyes. I couldn't feel my hands or feet. When they unstrapped me I jerked into a ball and my teeth clacked. Melissia burst into tears. The warm blankets felt heavenly. One patrol wiped my tears compassionately. Melissia hugged, kissed and cried over me, saying, "I love you, Mommy." Ray said, "Hi babe, I'm here. I love you." Lins loved over me. Eventually warm soup helped my temp rise. I heard the patrol whisper I'd reached a danger zone, nearing sleep, with rigid muscles. A few days later Melissia said tearfully, "I just realized I can't imagine what life would be like without you. I love you so much." God, TU for allowing this—I realize how much my family *and* I want me to live!

While sitting with Lins after school one day, I say, "I know most daughters pull away from their moms at a certain age. But Lins, I haven't had enough years. It can't be time yet!"

She laughs, saying, "It's time for me!" and we jostle playfully.

When Mel arrives from school Ray calls to talk with me, so she takes the phone, saying, "You can't talk to her. I get *my* four minutes with *my* mother first!"

He and I both laugh. Sometimes the "four minutes" Ray and I decided to carve out when he first gets home irritates her, now she throws it back on *him!*

One week later during a date with Melissia at the beach, after Ray tells the girls I need extra help when I'm tired, Melissia repeats the same thing as two years earlier about being glad to have a mom with MS. Then all happiness is obliterated. Ray says the girls' mom called, saying they'd told her I'm mean when he's not around, but they're afraid to tell him because he loves me. I ask them if that's true so I can apologize and change. They look surprised. Mel says she told her mom yesterday she was tired, and I'm hard on her and expect too much. This after she came home from school crabby and I held her lovingly!

Their mom also said it's inappropriate for me to tell them about the sexual abuse. It scares them. I ask if that's true, and Lins admits to being afraid when I cry but not for herself. Mel breaks into tears, saying she has nightmares after I've told them something. I feel terrible and ask their forgiveness tearfully, reaching to hold each one. I know I've been careful, but one time they were all tickling me I burst into tears, curled up, and went into a memory. I did explain it vaguely.

Sometimes when they see my tear-stained face after counseling they ask, "Was it hard, Mommy?" then put on a praise tape that we three dance to.

Oh God, I must never tell them anything though they show compassion.

Ray wants to know if they asked their mother to call.

Melissia answers, "Yes, because I want to live with my mommy."

Lins says she'd like to live both places, but she likes the influence we give her and she loves us. *God, am I to blame, or is it the ambivalence children of divorce feel?*

Ray states, "With all the wisdom I have I don't think this is the time for you to live there. Maybe someday, but not now."

After he leads us in a prayer that no one will feel like a prisoner, I begin fixing dinner. Each of the girls comes to me and I give them a long hug. They actually seem happy. As if Ray answered an unspoken question they toyed with.

Melissia asks cheerfully, "Mommy, when can you and I have another date?"

Matthew 16:24 says I must deny myself and pick up your cross if I'm to follow you. I lose my life by giving up the hope or right to not be criticized by the girls' mom. I am crucified with you and I should no longer live, but you through me (Galatians 2:20). TU for these circumstances, this pain you allow to help me grow.

Lins calls her mom after school, saying she had some misconceptions. "We're not having trouble with her. I didn't say that."

Her mom apologizes and asks Lins to tell me she's sorry and "Hi."

"Tell her I understand. She misses you and worries. It would be easy to suspect the worst."

One month later Melissia dials her mom after being angry with me.

When Ray asks what she said, Mel says, "I want to come live with you. Because Mommy has MS, she feels she can control this family, and I feel like I have to do too much."

My chest actually hurts as I sit folded over on the couch.

Ray says firmly but without anger, "You knew this woman had MS and would need help. We made a commitment. You are not to call your mother unless I'm home where I can hear. You've torn down this woman who loves you deeply!"

Melissia cries, "I'm sorry. I love you *so* much," several times.

"It hurt, but I accept your apology. Most kids have chores. I began making dinner when I was about eight, and my mom didn't have MS."

Lord, I know I don't control this family with MS. Help her see that.

In the morning Ray asks Lins to see her mom's latest letter. He reads her manipulation to keep working on him that they want to live with her. He tells Lins the enemy is trying to use her to break up our family.

At lunch Mel prays, "Help Mom see she can't break up this family."

I guess Lins told her.

I'm lying down while the rest of them are cleaning when Lins lies next to me, saying, "I love you so much. I don't ever want you to leave."

"I won't ever leave."

She continues, "We tell Mommy we miss her and want to be with her, and she says, 'Come live with me, tell your dad!'"

Then Melissia walks in, and I ask why she told her mom I control everything with MS. She says, "Well, it seems like you're lying around when we're working, and you could be working, too."

I explain, "Melissia, a person with MS must conserve energy because when it is spent, it's *gone*. Without resting there's nothing to go on, no reserve. I'm in tremendous pain at night because I overuse my muscles *every* evening. If I told you three how I *really* felt, you'd think I was whining. I'm not lazy."

I need to remember misunderstanding is common in families with MS *because we can look normal. I must educate them about various kinds of* MS *fatigue.* There's the overall kind due to demyelinated nerve fibers using more than normal energy to conduct impulses causing weakness and incoordination, the fatigue of stronger muscles trying to take over for weaker ones, plus normal muscle fatigue compounded by the disease itself.

A week after the last upheaval their mom's letter arrives. Ray reads it aloud and they both see her manipulation. Then he calls, asking how she'd like it if her other daughter had a parent to complain to.

"Jo is a fine woman and a good mother, and she really loves the girls. You feel guilty you abandoned them, and you can't handle that."

He points out the choices she made when she left them. She denies leaving the girls, only him, but he reiterates it was all three of them, and she made her own consequences that he even warned her of before she left. He says he wants the manipulation to stop.

She tells Melissia her daddy was mean. When Mel repeats that, I ask how *she* thought her daddy talked, and she answers, "Firmly, but truthfully, to get her to see what she's denying."

Lins says her mom apologized for putting pressure on them, and she's sorry she left them. Their daddy tried to tell her there would be consequences, and she wishes she'd considered them and guesses she's facing them now. She thinks it best they live with him for now and visit her. It would be better for their relationship; it might not be good otherwise.

It sounds like she's honest with Lins and manipulating Mel.

It's Lins' thirteenth birthday and she's asked me to go with her girl-friend and her mom to Disneyland. I squeal gleefully on the scary rides with Lins.

She says, "You're the best mom ever," hugging me.

I drawl, "Sure."

Lindsey's friend's mom, Julia, whispers, "It's not teasing—relish it."

Lins laughs, "We didn't even get stuck together like Daddy and us, we were magnetically drawn to each other!"

Julia pushes me around in a wheelchair with Lins occasionally sprawled on top. Our conversation about step-mothering affirms and comforts me as she admits she felt like giving up with her older step-daughter at times.

I find it difficult living here, especially now that I know I've scared the girls. I try to grieve silently, or sit in my car. The condo we're buying in order to build capital is so dark I feel even darker inside due to memories that still flash into realism at any time. I thank God for the stream and ducks and landscaping, and I pray to be satisfied when suddenly, someone knocks. Beve Samuelson, a realtor, asks if we're looking to sell and I say, laughing, "I wish!" I invite her in and bring the conversation around to my faith over the first of many cups of tea we share through the upcoming months.

Then I attend a seminar taught by a counselor and author specializing in sexual abuse. When we get to speak alone, I tell her Mom says MS is making me have delusions. She laughs sarcastically, saying a client's parents said mercury poisoning was affecting their daughter's mind! I express how guilty I can *still* feel for bringing up the incest, and she compassionately tells me she wishes I'd called her over two years ago. She would've assured me *not* to feel unjustified guilt, and that it can actually become a bondage to pray over. She also says MS might have to do with a "death wish" we should consider praying about. As I thank her, we hug warmly.

During counseling we pray that I'll be healed since I may have unwittingly made myself vulnerable to an illness—not that MS is psychosomatic. I just don't want to feel like years ago—that if I'm *not* healed, I don't have enough faith.

Free of MS. What would it be like? I want to be healed. *Do it, Lord, I trust you.* I'd love to have energy for you and Ray and the girls! If it's not your desire, keep me close in a humble walk of your strength in my weakness, and I commit to give you praise and show forth your grace and power.

After speaking for a mother/daughter banquet, I have my own wonderful Mother's Day. I'm taking Mel to school a couple days later when she says, "Do you mind if I call you 'Jo' again?"

"No, I'll love you the same. Are you mad?"

"No."

"Will you please tell me why later?"

"I can tell you now. I have a real mom, and it doesn't seem right to call you 'Mom' when I have a real mom alive."

I drop by my friend Jill's. As a counselor she encourages me to remember the issue is *not* my mothering, but Mel's stuff—her pain, confusion, and need for her mom causes anger at me. She urges me *not* to let Melissia change if she's angry. When I pick Mel up she hugs me and I say, "If it's better for you to call me 'Jo' I want you to do that. I won't love you any less." Throughout the day she calls me "Mommy," but I'm prepared to tell her next time she says "Jo," it can't be done out of anger.

I've reworked the letter Ray and I have discussed, and mailed it. On my birthday Mom calls to say, "Jo, I never said you had to recant everything above age four. I've never denied your father molested you." It feels like more crazy-making. I read 2 Corinthians 7:8–10:

"Even if I caused you sorrow by my letter, I do not regret it. Though I did regret it—I see that my letter hurt you, but only for a little while. Yet now I am happy, not because you were made sorry, but because your sorrow led you to repentance. For you became sorrowful as God intended and so were not harmed in any way by us ..." Abba, produce repentance in my family. I want them freed. I feel like a little girl who fell out of her family tree.

During the summer while the girls are gone, my neurologist says my shoulder pain is due to leaning on my crutches over ten years—a "sports injury"—the irony of trying to stay in shape! I pray the Norwegian physical therapist, Kirsten, can give me exercises for strengthening. I learn my right hip, neck and trunk are weak, and my trunk is also ataxic (out of balance and shaky). A friend seeing me in a swimsuit once said, "You've lost all your upper body musculature!" and the mirror seconded her opinion. Now I *know* the MS has progressed. Small facilitator muscles that control movement in the joints are weak, too, and my feet and arm pain are also MS related. Much of my pain is due to weakness affecting my posture—again, how ironic after Grandmother's constant instruction. Ray and I are both tearful to know Kirsten can help. We begin a sweet friendship renewed whenever I ask my neurologist for a referral to see her because I've become weaker.

Then the girls return. Melissia cries one night, "God gave me a family once and Mommy left. Now I'm afraid he'll take someone else away."

I hold her. "Melissia, we're not going to abandon you—you're not getting rid of me either."

Ray suggests we write a commitment in her Bible that we'll never leave her. We write in Lindsey's Bible as well, just as we did in both of ours.

New layers of memories continue to sap me, peeling away like an onion, making me cry burning tears of shame. I read Matthew 10:26—"So do not be afraid of them. There is nothing concealed that will not be disclosed, or hidden that will not be made known. What I tell you in the dark, speak in the daylight; what is whispered in your ear, proclaim from the roofs," and I know God is recalling memories up to heal me. I *still* pray to be truthful whenever ugliness knocks at my mind's door. I cry, "Cradle me, Abba, Daddy, cradle me in your love," and he does so tenderly. With each healed memory I know I'm becoming freer to be *me*—who God intended.

It's Sunday afternoon and *Western Union* calls. "Grandmother passed away September 30 at 8:25 a.m.————————family." My mouth agape, tears flow unchecked. I sputter it out to Ray and the girls and fall onto the couch. They surround me with comforting arms. I'd sensed all last week I should pray fervently for Grandmother but didn't call.

Lindsey says profoundly, "She's in heaven now, and she knows the truth."

I agree, startled, but thankful for her assessment. After weeping I lie down, drained from emotional exhaustion. Later we decide I should call to find out more.

Mom answers harshly, "Yes, Jo?"

"I received a telegram that Grandmother died. Could you tell me more?"

She softens slightly, "She hasn't been alert for months."

"I know. When I've called it was hard to communicate."

"About a week ago she decided to quit eating and went into a coma."

"I wish I'd known. I loved her very much. I would rather have been notified personally."

Mom retorts, "We all got together and decided to send the telegram. It would be less trouble. What is it that you want?"

"To be notified of the funeral arrangements."

She states, "Alright. Good-bye." I'm stunned.

It's as if the dream I had last week prepared me—I went *alone* to see Mom and Dad. She was scornful and Dad said angrily, "What are *you* doing here?" Now it's reality—they truly have shut me out. Ray said, "Their getting together to decide shows how sick the family is." Jill said, "It's sad and hard, but it's reality. The one who brings up the truth is cast out. You have another family." I think of Psalm 27:10–11 about if a father and mother forsake me you will not, Lord.

As I tell the group of ladies my family has totally rejected me for bringing up the incest, but I have a new family, and I'm part of *God's* family, I see amazement. I ask, "Would *you* like to be part of a family you'll never be rejected from?" and I see eagerness. Later I hear of several who've come into God's family and I'm overjoyed. I journal—"You *are* turning my wailing into dancing that my heart may sing and not be silent as Psalm 30:11–12 say. Hallelujah!"

One day I hear a preacher saying people misunderstand the Beatitude in Matthew 5:9—"Blessed are the peacemakers ..." because they assume it means we're to make peace with others at all cost. He says it means we are blessed because we show others how to have *real* peace with God, based on truth. He quotes Jesus in Luke 12:51–53—"Do you think I came to bring peace on earth? No, I tell you, but division. From now on ... they will be divided, father against son ... mother against daughter ..." I *know* I want my family to have the true peace of clear hearts before God.

Today Melissia's class welcomes me to speak about MS. I demonstrate my faulty coordination with a student holding his finger twelve inches from my face while I try to touch my finger between his finger and my nose, groping wildly through the air. The students gasp. I joke about messes with mascara and lipstick, then entertain questions. This begins an annual event in several classes, and I treasure their letters of appreciation.

A first-grade student raises his hand timidly to ask, "Does *anything* in your body work right?" and I burst out laughing. Now, whenever I'm told something is okay, I think *something in my body works right!*

I sit at my desk after Thanksgiving remembering seeing my neurologist just this week. I said with tears filling my eyes, "It's harder to sing well. Is it MS?" He gave me a fatherly hug, saying, "Yes. Your coordination is worse and singing takes that." I told Ray in the car I was so grateful he was there for me. I remembered Kirsten saying my attitude has made MS better for me than the bitter attitude of some of her patients. I write—"I take my vocal problems as a challenge. You gave me this talent. Until you take it away, I'll try to keep it strong and useful for your glory!"

On Christmas Melissia cries, "This was the best Christmas ever!" We ask why and she answers, "Well, because of my gifts and because of Daddy. He's never been very into it because of his childhood, and this year he's been really fun."

Lins adds, "And because we're together as a family."

We spend the evening with friends, where Ray tells about the time his family was broke, so they went into a Nazarene church that had gifts for underprivileged kids. Ray felt safe, as if someone cared. I sniff back tears as I look into others' shocked faces.

In the morning the leader of the Christian MS support group requests that I give a concert. He remembered my second annual holiday concert for the Orange County chapter of the National MS Society. I'm one of their peer-counselors, and as we talk he says, "Every time I see you walking with your crutches, I wonder if I hadn't given up when MS put me in a wheelchair if *I* would be walking today."

I say honestly, "You never know."

Girlfriends took me skiing yesterday and what fun we had! Today at PT I collapse into *total,* overall weakness. When I can finally move, it's only with vibrant shaking. In order to find a ride home, I call every friend whose number I carry until I reach someone, while another PT says, "I don't have *one* friend I could call!" I can barely make it onto the bed from the wheelchair. The girls comfort me, though they're a little scared. I call the church for meals, and other friends bring dinners. Though Ray's worried, I urge him to complete his out-of-town business. Each day I thank God for the precious help. What would we have done without their food and rides for the girls? What would I have done without these daughters? I'm so proud of how well we three handle the attack.

Mel says before I fly to Colorado to see friends the following month, "I'm glad you married Daddy. It's good to know you'll be together forever."

I state, "We will!" She says, "Don't go! Take me with you! Call every night!"

Each evening I hear how excited my family is to chase around looking for their hidden, inexpensive gifts. The envelope on the counter with a poem for each day explains where to search. I stay with the Clifts, and as I play on the floor with their infant, Doug, it feels like I'm discovering my lost childhood. Over lunch Judie Amen says to be with my family in denial would be rescuing them from responsibility and victimization for me. Peg says we cannot have a true relationship, so it's best not to relate. While

Anne and Dave and I ski, I feel like I'm in heaven soaring on eagle's wings, it's *such* a thrill. Then Ruth and Anne and I eat where Ray surprised me years before. It's a *good* trip.

When Lins speaks to me again with disrespect, I call Ray, and as I hand her the phone, I discover her under the table sucking her thumb. I pray for wisdom as I remember suggestions made by the counselor she's seeing, then I say, "Lins, I think there is a bigger reason for your nastiness. Can I hold you?"

She asks, "Why?"

"I just think there's more and you need to be held." We go to the couch and she cries so deeply it seems to rise from her toes. I say, "I love you. I'll never leave you," and her muffled cry is, "Why?"

So I tell her for at least ten minutes all the reasons I love her—who she is, how special, unique, sweet … She sobs through it all, then cries, "Why doesn't my mommy love me?"

All I can say is, "I don't know why she doesn't seem to show it."

Instead of Ray's assignment of writing many times "I will not be disrespectful," I have Lins write her feelings as I take Mel to gymnastics.

When I pick Lins up from her counseling appointment, she wants to know if I'd like to hear how she worked through her feelings. I answer, "Sure." Lins reads, "I took my anger out on Mommy (Jo) today, and all she did was tell me she loved me and would never leave me. I asked her why, and she told me all these things for a long time while she held me and I cried."

We look at each other with tear-soaked eyes. *Lord, TU for your wisdom. TU that Lins trusted me months ago, at her counselor's suggestion, to work through her feelings about the divorce with me. I've felt honored.*

On Mother's Day the girls appear with a tray-full of food to bring me breakfast in bed! After church my family takes me to a new store in the mall. The clothing is mostly pure white cotton with beautiful appliqués on them. *I get to pick one of these dresses!*

I look out at them from the dressing room with teary eyes, saying, "This is so special!"

Lins sighs, "I love your teary smiles."

When I put on the first dress I look in the mirror and say to myself *why, it's a pure little Jo. A pretty little girl!* I walk outside and Ray's eyes are also teary as he says softly, "That's just what I thought when I looked at that dress—you as a pure little girl untouched."

We hug and cry right there in the store as the girls smile.

Chapter 21

Taking Care of the Past So I Can Serve, Parent, and Comfort

I sit under the gazebo looking into a sea of faces at the Victorian Tea as our realtor, Beve, gazes back at me. After I sing my last song and lead them in a prayer Beve hugs me. Wiping her eyes, she says, "Ever since we met, God has been at work in my life. I became a Christian today!" *If we didn't live in our dark condo, I would never have met Beve!*

Ray says I'm so into my painful past as I write the book many have requested, I'm not lighthearted this summer.

It does unearth sadness like a backhoe. I've feared being truthful—maybe I'm not ready. I've also feared Ray will die and wonder *do I have to be an example in that, too?* You don't want me to live with irrational fear and worry—hyper-vigilance. Abba, you want me to be like a child at play. I must constantly re-parent my little child to keep from taking my mother's place as critical parent pushing undeserved guilt. Then I could truly love because I wouldn't be defensive. I hear, *"Cease striving to be perfect. Accept your weaknesses and rest in my power to surround you with my love."* TU, Abba. I want to live passionately, *not* fearfully!

We breathe in through our noses and out through our mouths to rid our muscles of lactic acid as Ray and I pump up a hill in the Orange County chapter's MS150 Bike Tour. Last week I worried I could harm myself by over-doing because my legs had weird buzzing sensations, but after praying I felt peaceful. My homemade hot pink fabric sign says "THANKS FOR RIDING, I HAVE MS"—becoming the source of numerous opportunities to share my faith. We lie around at a rest stop talking with other couples about how it's never wise to ride your tandem with unresolved issues because it's hard to get a rhythm on the bike, and we all chuckle! Ray affectionately calls me "wimp," "noodle," then "*gutsy* noodle" as I lie wiped out Monday.

> TU for the tears of pain, relief, and unabashed joy at the finish, though we were almost last. TU for the sheer pleasure of using my body—of not being paralyzed. For the praise songs we sang freely. That my sign, as well as my words of thanks on the bus impacted others according to the Society personnel. What a privilege!

Ten days later I hear from my neurologist the MS has progressed during the past three years. I thought so. I've been running into walls. Flattening my eye glasses. Poking fingers into Ray. I need to brace my hand in the way my great-aunt taught me to paint when I do fine-tuned things. My back goes out of alignment so frequently due to weakness, I'd have to *live* at a chiropractor's if one hadn't taught me how to adjust it on my own.

My doctor says, "If your name comes up in the lottery for the first FDA-approved-drug for MS—Betaseron—you should take it. It lessons the incidence and severity of MS attacks. If you find yourself sliding downhill, call me right away so we can begin steroids."

Does he expect that? I'm going to keep on skiing and biking with Ray and exercise to stay as fit as possible. I've been learning a new way of vocalizing to strengthen my voice. I am not giving in to MS!

A wise women's ministry director once told me, "You don't want to speak too much and be an absentee mom—those girls need you too much." I'm delighted they can be with me today when I say, "I'm so glad I didn't die when I tried to kill myself, or on the ski slope from hypothermia, because I get to tell you about Jesus!"

A woman whose eyes locked onto mine comes up afterwards, sobbing, "You stayed alive to tell *me!* My husband is a Christian, and wait till I tell him his prayer of years has been answered!"

Oh, Lord, I wish I could be a fly on the wall!

Melissia says as we head home, "I'm so glad I have you to myself! *My* mommy—all mine!" Roene smiles with delight at being a part of the experience *and* watching the girls love all over me.

Even after that, today has a bitter taste. I haven't spoken with Mom since Grandmother died, over fifteen months ago, though I've sent cards. I yearn at holidays for the impossible. I continue to pray, because I've read that holding out for a relationship based on truth is loving them with God's love (2 Thessalonians 3:14–15). My heart was right in confronting the incest, though my timing was definitely wrong. Proverbs 27:5–6 say—"Better is open rebuke than hidden love. Wounds from a friend can be trusted, but an enemy multiplies kisses." I know I acted in love because loving them means hoping for their repentance. "Love must be sincere. Hate what is evil; cling to what is good" (Romans 12:9). This means hope for the best in my family though I hate the wrong done to me. I *want* to be reconciled with them.

After chatting with a friend, I realize as I've faced difficulties God's revealed more truth, showing me who I really am and who he wants me to be.

Oh Abba, you *are* revealing more truth and I'm so sad. Lindsey told me as we drove home, "You're always, at least most of the time, angry at Mel and me. And you use swear words!" I was shocked. I told all three of them later, "I'm *so* sorry. I don't want to be like that, I want to be like Jesus. Please, will you forgive me?" Lord, I plead with you to end the memories.

Though we haven't seen him for some time, I called our counselor two months ago because I still experience too much fear. I put off counseling because Inga and Ruben are in the U.S., on their way here.

Melissia says, "This is so exciting!"

Inga asks while the girls are in school, "How is it with your family?" and tears flow down my cheeks as I curl up against her. "You are as my daughter, Jo. Let go of them."

We have a fun five days then Inga holds Melissia, saying, "You are my granddaughter. We are three adopted generations." Inga hugs Lindsey good-bye lovingly while Lins says, "See you next time in Sweden," grinning.

I cry as I put them on the train, tears of gratitude for the way they loved my family, and Inga's mothering my hurting child within.

Now we need to deal with Lindsey's increasing rebellion since both Ray and I see enormous potential problems. Ray asks, "Why aren't you tougher with her?"

I answer, "Every time I am, I get this withdrawal-of-love-routine and I'm sick of it!"

Ray told me I have a vindictive spirit against Lins and I agreed—even though I don't want to. I love Lins, but I need to be mature enough to *not need her love.* She's an angry little girl who can be abusive. I hurt for her, but also my little Jo who is triggered to feel unloved. Frankly, when she says certain things I feel like the child! I don't know how to parent well. I must depend on *your* power to love when I'm bankrupt. The problem is Lins' untrustworthiness. She says it's all us, not her, and she can be very intimidating.

Then I hear on a Christian counseling program that people who try to control others are really trying to control their own emotions that are out of control. To break out of feeling controlled or manipulated, I need to realize what I want—approval? To not be left out? Then I need to tell myself I *don't* need that. Being a pleaser was and is controlling because it means I'm trying to prevent being abandoned, to make sure I'm loved. Every time I sense irrational anger, I need to ask why—it shows pain from the past is rearing its ugly head and needs to be dealt with in order to be decapitated.

Now I'm experiencing such weakness I lie in bed, praying the flare-up will not prevent me from speaking. When I'm able to walk, holding tightly onto walls, I cheer! And when I sit on my stool in the Catholic parish, I tell how I felt *just last week,* giving God all the glory. Men along with women cry as I tell about Ray's growth. A woman phones to convey her husband is hearing from men who were touched to know *they* need to admit and experience anger hidden inside to keep from dumping it on their families. *Abba, what a privilege to know what we've gone through can jumpstart growth in women* and *men.*

We run (well, I try) from room to room in our new home. Beve sold our condo and located this new townhouse closer to the ocean, just up the hill from a new high school. The girls grin from ear to ear in their own rooms. I grin because of how cheerfully bright it is.

Someday I know my whole life will be this bright. I work for months on memories so thick and deep, a layer of onion so pungent, I fear I'll be swallowed up in stinging tears that will never end. A new memory makes my heart jump into my throat and I can't breathe. This species of panic must be controlled for me to be congenial.

When Ray tells me on our next date he's been angry with God for allowing me to be abused as a child, I see how it's played out in his life lately. He finds it amazing I have such a good relationship with the Lord, and I say it must be his grace. I pray, "Help Ray accept life as it is, to love you, and know your love."

After church we go to Chili's for late lunch. Mel has told me, "Happy Mother's Day" over and over again, with, "I love you soooo much," as has Lins. Ray asks them, "What thing have you appreciated about Mommy in the past few months?"

Mel says, "That I can talk to her anytime. That she's there for me."

How precious. I told her I always want to be approachable, not for her to worry about interrupting my naps because I snapped at her before.

Lins says, "That she's been patient with my schedule and me, and not nagging me a lot; and she's picked me up several times and brought me home."

Wow! That's just what I've been praying for and working on. TU *Lord, I really needed this!*

When I ask Ray what he appreciates he answers, "The way you protect the girls and stand up to me."

I'm stunned because my silent cue that Ray was too intense didn't work, and I *know* Mel is—she couldn't sleep because of our argument last weekend! I say, "But you've been angry at me—"

He says, "Well, I realize they *need* your protection—it's usually *my* problem."

I laugh, saying, "They need you to protect them from *my* dysfunction and me to protect them from yours. What would it have been like if our parents protected us?"

As we all talk about this, I say, "I'm so blessed to have you," and Ray says, "That's good, 'cause you're stuck with us!"

One evening Lins hands me the phone while we're eating, mouthing *somebody who's rude!* I say, "Hello," and hear my sister tell me in a controlling tone she didn't know how to get hold of me. I could've said the Christmas cards I sent came back with "moved," but instead listen as she tells me Dad died yesterday.

"Thank you for letting me know."

She says the memorial service will be tomorrow. My family offers to stay home, but I encourage Ray to drive the girls to church youth group while I ask myself how I feel. I've grieved the loss of Dad for years. I've grieved the loss of a *loving* dad, as well.

I do *not* cry.

When Ray leaves town for five days I find a card in my underwear drawer that says—"If it hurts you to look back, frightens you to look ahead, then just look beside you ... I'll be there." He added—"*Always,* Love, Me." I faithfully give him a card whenever he leaves town, and he gives me one with *just* what I need to hear.

As if the basement of my mind was never before completely cleaned, memories vomit forth. I shake with the horror of some, wail with the pain of most, and sob with the shame of all. I was abused from preschool until, as a senior, I escaped Dad's grasp and ran down the sidewalk chanting the same thing Mom told me as a child—"It was just a nightmare." The nightmare is revealed when I read Marilyn Van Derbur's account in *People Weekly*,[24] trembling and sobbing uncontrollably. I *know* Dad came into my room and raped me often at night. Then mom appeared and rubbed my back tenderly, saying, "It was just a nightmare, Jo." *Did she know?*

Today our counselor says, "You have soared, and you will again. You have oil on your wings, but we'll clean it off and you'll fly again." I leave his office reminding myself so I'm ready for my family—a victor—not a victim.

While the girls are with their mom for the summer, Ray and I take the ferry to San Juan Island, northwest of Seattle. In the morning we board a two-man kayak to join a group leaving Roche Harbor. I sit in the back because the strongest person is to paddle vigorously in front. The problem is, the person in the rear has their two feet on pedals controlling the rudder that turns the kayak. I'm supposed to paddle a certain way while I man the rudder in the opposite direction with *my* coordination? We turn in circles and Ray loses his cool as the group heads out far into the harbor. I yell, "I'm trying!" A couple from the group stop by our table at breakfast the next morning to say how great they think it is I even *tried* to kayak with MS. From now on every time we see a kayak Ray and I joke, "We should get one of those," knowing it's the exact thing we should *not* do! As we take a cruiser into the strait, I go down to the head below deck, only to miss a huge Orca whale breach over the bow of our boat! So we begin teasing about my missing things due to my pit stops. But I *don't* miss watching about fifty Orcas cavort and play for us from two of the three resident pods in the area—they're amazing!

Then Lins calls from her mom's, distraught, wanting to come home early. Ray changes her flight, and while he goes to San Francisco for the dental meeting at which I planned to join him, I'm home comforting Lins, while praying for wisdom. The girls' mom calls in tears, saying a detective is on "the case about Lins," so I call the involved neighbor who says there never was a case, *or* a detective. When I speak with their mom in a few minutes, she tells me she said that just to make Lins take responsibility! Lins feels like her mom wants to ruin her life. Ray and I aren't sure what *really* happened, but we know it's being handled incorrectly.

Melissia returns, calling me "Jo," and I tell her that's fine if it's an adjustment time like usual, or if she wants to change, but it can't be because she's angry at me, wanting to hurt me. Mel says it's just adjusting, though she did change it to hurt me before. I'm thrilled to share my feelings calmly with her.

But the days are stressful, with Melissia and Lindsey arguing more. Their mom calls only Mel. I tell her what their mom said to me about the detective so she knows the truth. This thing between their mom and Lins is dividing our family. Ray and I pray.

It's October and Mel lies on our bed, saying, "I'd like to call you Jo now. I don't feel comfortable calling you Mom."

"You have that right, but after five years I'd like to know why."

"I don't know."

"Has your mom asked if you're still calling me that?"

"I honestly don't remember, but my step-dad says he's against it." I ask if it's because I've been honest about her mom regarding Lins, but she says, "No, I was thinking about it before."

"Sweetie, you gave me a gift five years ago and now you're taking it away. I love you just as before, but I can't say I'll respond the same until I get used to it. I'm not angry, just hurt."

Mel's face falls, "I don't want to hurt anyone."

She leaves our room and I feel so sad. Yet, I don't want Mel to feel badly. I knock on her door and hold her in my arms as I say, "I love you," stroking her back while she cries. "I'll be here in the morning," I say, and she sobs more.

She looks me in the eye, "I love you very much," and I repeat those words.

I cry until 1:00 a.m. because it's so unfair the girls have such trauma to deal with, and I feel I've lost a family member—Melissia. I know it's not true, it just feels like it. My family's rejection must be surfacing through this.

When Mel gets home from school she says, "I miss Mommy so much every night that it's hard to call you Mom in the morning. I have thought about changing what I call you for a month, but once I did it I felt sad. I cried most of the night. I think I made a mistake. I need to be able to call you Mom when I come home from school. I'd like to call Mom and tell her I *want* to call you that, but I'm afraid of what my step-dad will say."

I tilt my head, "Maybe you don't need to say anything."

She says, "I feel like I lead two lives."

"You missed God's ideal for the family and I'm sorry. So did I. You know, I called Ron's mother Mama all these years, even after he left me, because she's like a mom. Maybe you could tell yourself it's okay to have two moms."

She seems happy, like her old self.

In a few days Ray and I stand at the start of the MS150 at Newport Dunes where I take the megaphone and thank hundreds of riders lined up. We're again thrilled to make the ride. Like last year, we've trained for months, riding along the coast where it's coolest during the summer. Besides savoring opportunities to talk about our faith, I have the privilege of being interviewed by the *Orange County Register* newspaper, as well as writing a thank you letter to riders for the next Orange County chapter newsletter. I'm overwhelmed when they honor me with their local annual MS Achievement Award.

For awhile Ray's been attending a group with men whose wives have suffered similar trauma to mine. He tells me he shared his feelings of anger and unfairness that we have to deal with it. Then he said, "Knowing all I know now, I would marry Jo again. She's brought so much meaning into my life."

Another said, "That's a testimony of your love for Jo."

Then Ray says, "Only recently, I've felt loved by God no matter *what* I do."

I cry, "I've been praying that for you for years—it's in my prayer journal!"

"*Really?*" he asks, smiling.

I write—"PTL! No wonder I see his love for you growing!"

We four still have meals together that amaze their girlfriends whose families don't bother with that, but our family life isn't what it was a year ago. Ray and I realize, for one thing, the girls are growing up. But most of it revolves around Lins being abandoned again by her mom. Mel went to see her at Christmas *without* Lins. Mel receives letters and cards. Lins does not. Our hearts break when we hear from the school she's having difficulty. And though parents of divorce are *not* to speak ill of the other parent to the children, Ray and I feel we have no choice but to point out (though I try to do it less than he) what their mother is doing is wrong, and Mel feels guilty for receiving things when Lins doesn't.

One evening Melissia and I stand alone in the kitchen, and since I haven't heard from Mom for years, she says, "I can't imagine a mother treating her daughter like yours does you."

It's as if she's wearing blinders. I feel like saying *your own mother is treating your sister the same!* Instead, I add, "I can't either, Melissia," and hug her for feeling compassion. It's not often I sense it from her.

At times it feels like I've been deleted from her consciousness like an unwanted word. Ray and I believe, as do friends who are counselors, that she's transferring to me the anger she cannot put on her mom because she has to make her mother "good." So that means *I* am *bad*.

As I prepare to speak by request on "Spirit Power," I claim Colossians 1:9–12—"That *I* would live a life worthy of *you* and please *you* in every way, bearing fruit in this work as *I* grow in the knowledge of God and am strengthened with *Your* power so that *I* may have great endurance and patience, joyfully giving thanks to my Abba!"

After my talks, while celebrating the Lord's Supper, the pastor anoints me with oil, saying, "God has given me a new name for you Jo. It is 'Joy.' I see the work God is doing through you."

I pray silently, *The ministry you've given me* is *joyful. TU for the joy set before me of being your servant. Hallelujah!*

One note I receive moistens my eyes—"Most speakers challenge me to return home and 'change,' but you gave the 'secret' to change—the powerful Holy Spirit who lives within me!"

All glory to you, Spirit!

I'm experiencing such emotional healing, when I sing "I've Just Seen Jesus" on Easter morning and people compliment me later, I ask, "But, did you see *Jesus? That's* what I wanted for you. *That's* what I prayed for!" because it's as if *I* saw him.

Mel will be going to Colorado *without* Lins this summer. As I've shared my hurt for Lins, two girlfriends suggest *I* take her to Sweden, confirming what my mind has already pondered! Before I can complete my reasoning about wanting to show Lins how special and loved she is, Ray proclaims, "I want you to take her!"

I go around Ray's desk and kiss and hug him fiercely, saying, "The girls say when I'm away you become depressed. You have to promise me you won't do that."

"There will be some rough times because you're the most important thing in the world to me, but I'll try."

Later, I pull Lins aside. "I asked Daddy if I could take you to Sweden this summer. Would you like to go?"

Her eyes bulge. In an ecstatic voice she cries, "Oh, yes! I can't believe it! I wanted to go *so* much. *Now,* I'm happy!"

"I wanted you to have something to look forward to like Melissia."

When Lins tells Melissia, she says, "That's neat. Well, I'll go later with Dad. Just me and my dad!"

I explain to her I want to take Lins because she isn't going to see their mom, and she'll feel bad, *not* because I don't want to take Mel.

On Mother's Day Lins hands me a homemade card with the form of a bunny cut out of black construction paper so the pink paper beneath colors his body, saying:

"Dear Mom, Mothers Day is a day to express ... I love you so much. I was blessed with a terrific velveteen mom. And that's more than any child could ask. I know it's hard. I'm not always the easiest person to get along with. But you're doing a great job. Keep up the good work (and report to me when you're done. HA, HA.) You are awesome. I love you, Lins" (Then she quotes from the book how the rabbit becomes real from the story I so loved her reading to me years ago, *The Velveteen Rabbit*).

Both Lindsey and I have tear-filled eyes as I hug her tightly while thanking her.

Ray, who hasn't been totally alone for years, is so lonely while Lins and I visit Sweden, we talk frequently. I wrote ahead to my friends, and they're especially loving and sensitive to Lindsey. Inga and Ruben treat her as their grandchild, and they take us to various parts of the country where my friends now live, as well as parts to which I've never been. Though I want this to bless our relationship, Lins is distant. She feels angry, but hurt also haunts her very existence like a nagging pain one can't get rid of. It isn't until after we return home that she talks about the fun she had.

As I compare this trip to mine alone in 1985, I realize I *knew* God wanted to bless me! I see that back then I felt unworthy and needed assurance my friends still loved and accepted me, though I was divorced. This time I saw us as equals—in need of God's grace—who love others with *his* love. As I shared privately about my memories, I saw only belief and compassion. I felt safe with them and so glad we could be open with one another.

It's our anniversary and Ray takes me to Cannon's overlooking Dana Point Harbor. As the maitre d' leads us, I spy a vase of roses on a table next to the window. I think *surely those roses aren't for me,* seeing another empty table. But we continue walking right to them! Ray had a florist deliver to the restaurant, to be placed on a window table, the vase hugging six red roses, one for each year! I give him a big kiss in front of everyone, and he holds me close. Romance fills our hearts as the full moon rises over the harbor glistening with sunset hues.

I exclaim, "I don't believe anything is perfect, but *this is!*"

"It means a lot that you feel so happy about it."

Through wet eyes I smile, "The roses, for all to see, make me *know* you're proud of me."

He says, teary-eyed, "I am. I want everyone to see that I love *you*."

We reminisce about our marriage—the hard work and how it's paying off.

The MS150 is much more difficult for me to recover from this year. I wilt like a spinach leaf in a skillet, causing more stops where we literally pour gallons of water over me as steam seems to rises off my overheated body. We can't complete the distance, taking a sag-wagon for a few miles. I begin exceptionally tired the second day and lie on sidewalks to adjust my back. But I wear my sign and encourage the riders like always. Other people who have MS hold homemade signs this year expressing their thanks.

Then our pastor tells about their family's desire to have an artist sketch portraits of their daughters, but the girls felt uncomfortable around him, as did his wife, so they cancelled the appointment. They discovered recently he'd been prosecuted as a pedophile child molester. They're so grateful God protected their girls. Inside I cry *Why didn't you protect me, God?*

At home I tell Ray how I felt, and he responds, "God did something different in protecting you. He kept you from remembering until now, and he kept you for him. And I've come to believe that those who've been hurt deeply have deeper relationships with God."

My eyes wide, I cry, "I agree! I've loved God so much."

Ray continues, "And God does use it for good if we let him."

I sigh, "Do you realize you are past the anger-at-God stage where you cried it isn't fair?"

He states, "It *isn't* fair."

"I know, but you know it and can now trust God with it instead of feel angry. I hear and see healing in you!"

He cries, "You're right!" and we grin happily.

It's February. Ray has just asked me out on a date for tonight and I accepted. Mel is at the stairs bottom yelling for Lins to hurry up. Ray stands about a yard away from me.

"Tux! No, you don't!" I call as our cat dashes at me. A quick deep-knee bend and I can catch him! My hands grab wildly for Tux, (who looks like he wears a tuxedo coat and white gloves). I feel his body, then his tail slip through my fingers as he tears down the steep flight of stairs—and I tumble headfirst after him, thump after painful thump.

My head snaps all the way back, then forward to my chest. I land at the bottom of the stairs upside down. I can feel *nothing* below the excruciating pain in my neck.

"God, help me!" I shout.

Chapter 22

Overcoming Near Paralysis to Fight in the Trenches

Immediately, I feel searing pain from my shoulders to my fingers. My legs tingle. *I'm not paralyzed.* "Thank you, Jesus!" I cry.

Ray, seeing me fall, yells, "Lindsey, call 911! Then call the church for prayer." Melissia looks at me in horror.

Our neighbor who is a nurse suddenly appears, having heard the commotion.

"Lisa, help me move—my neck *hurts.*"

"No, Jo. It's too dangerous."

Standing above my contorted body sprawled up the stairs, Ray whispers, "I love you, baby."

When the ambulance crew arrives one reaches to straighten me and Lisa grabs the neck stabilizer from another. "Don't you dare move her before putting this on first!" Lisa attaches the collar, then moves away.

In the emergency room a nurse grasps my hand, but I yank it back.

Ray growls, "She has burning pain. Don't touch her!" I can't even bear a sheet on me. Lins and Melissia look on fearfully, then each tells me they love me, kissing my forehead.

"Baby," I say, "I'm sorry. That was so stupid to reach for Tux."

Ray responds, "Don't ever say that again. It was just a reflex." Now I really cry because I am *not* to blame for this fiasco.

In intensive care a neurosurgeon explains my cervical spinal cord injury at C5/C6 where my disk protrudes into the spinal cord with bruising elsewhere.

I whisper, "I love God and know I'm in his hands."

"It's obvious God still wants you here or you wouldn't be," the surgeon replies.

They almost moved me without the neck collar—the disk could've severed the cord—Lisa was your emissary, Lord!

The rehabilitation specialist adds, "You're very lucky. I've seen people paralyzed from this type of fall." *Oh, TU God!*

I know how it feels to be so weak because of MS I can't walk, but my legs do not want to move. *Think, Jo. Tell them to move one inch at a time! God, please help me!* Tears fill my eyes as fatigue engulfs me. The neurosurgeon said the fullest recovery prognosis depends upon early, intensive rehabilitation—I need visual motivation.

At my request the family picks out photos I tape into a collage—one of us four; one of Ray and me riding our tandem; another of me swishing down a slope. When I ask how soon I can ski my doctor says, "Jo, this type of injury typically takes two years to heal completely. Besides, skiing is dangerous!" I've skied at least part of every season for ten years, even if that took rehabilitating after MS relapses. I want to ski again!

One nurse says, "I should just encourage you—but how do you do it—MS, now this?"

I answer, "Frankly, without God's help, I might give up."

She brings ice cream to my room at night so I can tell her about God.

Each morning, after calling the girls to say, "Have a good day. I love you," I listen to Mel's praise tape. Nurses say, "The other patients love your music." Then Ray arrives with cappuccino and a kiss on his way to work. I smile in his love. A PT wheels me to therapy where I roll ever-so-slowly from side-to-side while wearing my stiff neck collar. I learn to stand, shaking with weakness. Then I drag one foot forward, toe-first, followed by the other a couple steps and sit down. I eagerly tell my therapists that God loves them, and how he'll use this in my life if I let him.

Every lunch-hour Ray visits, and every evening after the girls fix dinner with one of my recipes, he reclines beside me. He says, "I have to know you're all right, to be with you," and I know his reason is *love,* not dependency. Then I tell the girls good night. I'm proud that they've continued grocery shopping, making a menu first like I taught them. I pray God uses this in *each* of our lives.

Long ago I learned the axiom, "No pain—no gain" from PTs—I had *no* idea. Before the OT, I warily push my hands into bowls of raw rice, crying out, tears spilling over my cheeks! My "homework" to reduce the severe hypersensitivity consists of rubbing my hands and arms with a soft piece of cloth, working up to stiff cardboard. This searing pain triggers a stomach-ache, so I rub while concentrating on TV or a friend. Tonight Jill visits and we compare the desensitizing of physical pain to the scraping out of infectious sorrow by reliving of memories.

A few weeks into therapy a vice of MS fatigue clamps me to the bed. Fear and discouragement blast my peace.

> God, you alone see the big picture. This isn't merely about my body needing healing. This is about suffering producing perseverance; perseverance, character; and character, hope like Romans 5:3–4 say. I count this joy, Lord. If I wasn't here nurses wouldn't have purchased tapes to share with friends and listen to in their cars! Trisha said, "We're all being touched by you." I sense your presence filling all the dark spaces with your warm, sweet love. You give me joy every morning. Great *is* your faithfulness, but I'm scared I won't even walk like I did. I'm so buzzed with IV-Solumedrol steroids I feel I could blast into space. Please heal me.

Since I don't recover from the attack enough to continue therapy, I'm to be moved to my neurologist's hospital for further treatment. Nurses and PTs and OTs hug me, saying, "We'll miss you!" and *all* of us cry.

The ambulance crew rolls me up to the new hospital room, but before

I can even say thanks, a nurse begins taking off my sweat pants and panties in front of them! *This time* I speak up.

"I think it would have been respectful to wait!"

"We'll be putting in an IV and ..."

I reiterate how I feel and she apologizes. *I stood up for myself!*

When I finally arrive home, Melissia hugs me from behind the wheelchair, saying, "I'm glad you're here. I missed you."

I tear up and say the same. After asking for meals from the church, I realize I'm denying the girls the privilege of cooking for me. I apologize and pray they're blessed, and when we sit to eat I say, "I really missed this!"

Ray's keeping his promise to my neurologist to take vacation to help me with each faltering step, holding onto the stabilization belt around my waist as I lean on a walker while wearing the stiff neck collar. I feel immensely grateful to walk, however slowly. Ray says he enjoys caring for me, even helping me to the bathroom, and I tear up. Tears pour actually, due to steroid build-up.

Tonight he asks Lindsey to pick up something from the store. When she returns I realize how crabby I am, so I pray silently, *God, search my heart* ... then say, "Lins, I'm ashamed to admit I'm jealous that you can drive and I can't! Please forgive me."

She hugs me. "Sure, Mom. I'm sorry you can't drive."

Later, Mel helps me onto the shower stool. "Be careful! Isn't it kinda scary that you almost died?"

I respond, "Yes, scary *and* exciting because God says it isn't my time yet!" Later, she calls from her friend's to tell me she loves me. I cherish the moment.

In several weeks, just as walking becomes slightly easier, a lead anchor seems to hang from my waist landing me back in my wheelchair. Evidently the Betaseron I've been injecting every other night hasn't taken effect yet. I write—"I feel sad not being productive, but I must remember I'm significant *because you love me* and Jesus proved that on the cross. I can live for you, God, even if I can't do much. I can still praise you."

Lins prays at dinner, "Mom would not get too discouraged she's not getting better as fast as she wants. Help us to encourage her and show compassion." Ray squeezes my hand as I thank her.

As soon as the attack lifts, after *more* Solu-medrol, my home-health-care PT returns. One labored footstep at a time, I recover the ability to walk with my cool-aids. Then in a month, my legs feel as if they weigh tons *again*. Ray holds me as I cry, exhausted and sad to be experiencing yet *another* exacerbation which threatens my recovery. I can't even take steroids, I've reached my limit.

Ray asks, "Are you scared you won't regain your strength and abilities?" Tears run down my face as I nod. "Well, we'll just have to change our life-style and have fun anyway."

I sniff, "As long as I have you."

He kisses me and says, "You do."

Ray has proven himself through this. His tenderness grows like a garden fertilized by suffering as he calls me sweet names, saying I look attractive when I feel the opposite!

I whisper through tears, "I will still praise God." As I praise God because he *is* God, it's as if I see my fear flying away.

TU, Lord, for Ray's calming effect. I praise and thank you for your love. I *can trust you.* I'm in your hands, you're in control. Ray told Don this week, (whose wife has MS, and who advised Ray against dating me) he has *never* regretted marrying me. TU even for hair loss due to the steroids. I count it all joy through my tears!

Amazingly, a month later I can walk slowly down a sidewalk in Vail, Colorado, with Ray at a sales meeting. We left Lins with the Peters' while Mel is with their mom. When we try to rent a tandem, the manager looks dubious since I'm using crutches and wear a neck collar, relenting only when we sign a consent form. During the short ride through Vail Valley, with towering peaks reflecting the spirit of hope God's given us, Ray and I decide to train diligently for the upcoming MS150. As we drive back to the Peters' we sight a herd of elk, mountain sheep and goats. We're thrilled, but even more so because Lindsey's mom apologized for how she's treated Lins these past two years! At seventeen, she *needed* this.

Eight months after my "stair-dive" as Ray calls it, I tell bikers through a megaphone about God healing my spinal cord injury so we could ride. Many approach us about how that affected them. These are *tough* miles. It's so hard and "hurts so good," and I'm soooo exhausted. Yet I feel overwhelming joy that God chose to spare me from death or paralysis and gave me patience with my painful neck to train. "I give you all the glory, Lord!"

Melissia and I struggle off and on, as do Lins and I. Then I remember Ruth telling me she and her daughter have difficulties. Mother/daughter relationships go through changes at this age.

When I ask Mel if she'd like to run the sound equipment for me she says, "I'll do it! I can learn!" She proves to be an expert, saying, "It was my gift. I'm proud of you."

While Mel and I talk to sixth-graders about MS, she's asked how she feels about me having it. Mel says, "I don't really mind. When I was in fourth grade a friend said, 'You have a handicapped mom, don't you hate her?' I couldn't understand that—why would I hate someone just because they're handicapped? Besides, I've learned a lot having a mom who's disabled. It helps me with other people. When she can't walk and is in bed, sure, it's not fun to have to bring her water and stuff, but I think, 'What if it was me?'"

On Thanksgiving morning Melissia walks into the kitchen saying, "I was thinking if you'd died last year things would be very different. I'm thankful for you."

After dinner with the Lettows, Mel acts the opposite, calling me "she." Ray asks, "What do you want to call Mom?"

Mel explains since she's gotten closer to her mom, she feels she only has one, but I talked her out of it when she brought up "Jo" last time. I say that's not how I remember it—after telling me she wanted to change, she said she'd made a mistake. I explained about my mother-in-law, Mama, and she seemed peaceful.

"Mel, I've felt your anger building for the past two years." *Since your mom rejected Lins.* "I don't think I deserve it. I didn't break up your family. I know it's been hard on you having a step-mom. I've cried for you. It hasn't been easy for me either. But if I knew everything would happen just the same, I would marry your dad all over again. The joys have outweighed the hurts."

Mel states, "They don't for me."

"Feel free to call me 'Jo.'" I walk past the bathroom where Lins stares in the mirror and say, crying, "Mel wants to call me Jo. If you want to also, I'll understand."

Lins looks at me with her eyes scrunched together.

I pray to let go of the hurt, able to hear Mel call me "Jo." I praise you through tears that cloud my vision. TU for allowing this. What have I been doing for seven and a half years? I feel my velveteen mom status stripped by Mel. Use this to break me further. I don't need the title of "Mom." Shine through me with your love.

Ray tells me in the morning he's been so hurt by Melissia that he cried with a man at the men's retreat. He says, "Some families *never* blend."

I cry, "I thought we had—that's what hurts!"

He sighs, "We did. This is another season. Don't let this ruin the happy memories you've got of our times together and yours with the girls. I think you've done a good job—leave her to God. Melissia has all we gave her, and we need to let her make her own choices. I think if she wants to stay in Colorado, I'll let her."

After I ask Mel to help me decorate for Christmas she calls me "Mom," but in the morning she's angry. Melissia says, "I ask God every night for forgiveness for the way I treat you, but I think he's quit forgiving me because I do it day after day. I hate waking up because it starts all over again. I ask God to take me in my sleep so I won't wake up."

I touch her hand and say, "That concerns me. Maybe you should talk with someone."

"I couldn't talk to somebody."

"Then write down your feelings about me to God."

She cries, "I don't want to show you love because that means I have to have a new family!"

"We've been a family for over *seven* years! Your dad raised you *alone* for seven years before that. *You have two families!* Have you considered staying with your mom?"

"I have, but that would be running from the problem."

Mel is sobbing, so I ask if she wants to be held. She nods and I pull her into my arms, saying I love her and God forgives us whenever we ask. I pray for her to deal with her feelings so she no longer wants to die.

She sniffs, "I think I would do better if I could talk to you and Dad like this."

Later, Ray says, "I doubt she'll receive anything from me because she just doesn't want to accept the reason for her second mother is because *her first mother left.*"

Since Lins still calls me "Mom" I ask Ray whether he's going to call me "Mom" or "Jo" to the girls now and he just shrugs sadly, "I don't know."

Our family is privileged *once again* to see a neighbor become a Christian! Teri's been going to church with us, and today she realizes she needs Jesus in her life. I cry tears of joy. Two weeks later I meet an MS peer-counselee for lunch at Chili's Restaurant, thinking she wants to talk about multiple sclerosis. Instead, she says, "What I really want is to get closer to God," and Debbie prays right there to know Christ! These two coming to Jesus are *wonderful* Christmas presents.

Both girls go to their mom's this year, and after Ray and I spend a quiet Christmas he prays with me. I've prepared myself by writing out possible scenarios so I'm ready, since Mom hasn't contacted me in years, though I've continued sending cards.

"Hi, Mom, this is Jo."

"Jo, who?"

"Your daughter."

"You don't sound like Jo," she says, with sincere confusion. Then her voice cracks with emotion, "I love you, Jo."

"I called to see how you are."

"I'm doing good. I can hardly believe it's you, it's been so long. You've been in my prayers every day."

I say, "Thank you."

She cries, "I'm so tickled to hear from you."

I ask about her health and the family, then she says, "Thank you for calling."

I rub the bed comforter as I say, "I love you," and she repeats it.

After pondering the conversation I journal—"I'm glad I called. I believe I was filled with you, Spirit. I'm surprised she was so appreciative. Work in her heart through my call."

When the girls return, Lindsey says she gets angry if she sees *the look* on my face when Mel calls me "Jo." *God, you know I don't always handle it well. Help!* Lins says Mel never wants to hear me speak because I lie about how great our family is. *God, is my ministry a sham? Should I give it up? Mel told me just a few months ago after hearing me she was proud.*

I ask how Lins feels. "Sometimes it's so touching I want to cry, but I'm closer to you." Lins says things go well for a few days then I'm just like I was, so mean, like during the memories.

"I'm so sorry I took anger out on you then and now. I make mistakes and ask forgiveness. Children of divorce have an advantage—when things aren't going well they can say, 'I'd rather live with the other parent.' I'm very sorry and *will* try to change, Lins."

We hug warmly and I *know* I'm not a failure. I must remember friends tell us biological parents express irrational anger, as well, and must apologize.

You gave me this privilege and thorn (2 Corinthians 12:7) of step-mothering to make me more Christ-like and to bless the girls. When I react to Mel saying my name, rather than let it be as natural as hearing "Mom," I put on her the same pressure that *her* mom has for years, and I'm no different. I need you so much.

While Mel and I are watching TV in the evening, knowing I feel totally to blame I say, "I don't want you to move in August."

She says, "I know."

I continue, "I've shown happiness because I want *you* at peace, happy. You're always welcome back here."

Mel says, "Thank you."

"I intended on taking you on a trip, but with my stair-dive, I didn't see how I could." My eyes are filling with tears.

"I know. I love you," Mel says as she comes over and hugs me. "I love you, too," I say tearfully.

On Mother's Day I say into her recorder, "Hi Mom, this is Jo …" When my birthday arrives I cry, "I wish she would call," knowing little Jo will always want her.

Ray's flying home and I wonder *should I drive by airport-pick-up like he expects, or hide behind the post at his terminal and surprise him?* Heading to the car I miss the bottom step, then hear a crunching sound accompanied by sharp pain. Though I'm grateful it's not my head or neck, I whine, "God, I wanted to ride in the MS150!" I page Ray to take a cab. The orthopedist says, "It will take three months to heal." I respond, "Then it will be fine for ski season," because I'm thinking February—two years since my "stair-dive." In a week Ray pushes me, with my aqua cast, in my wheelchair to the starting line so I can encourage the riders through the sound system as I sniff back tears.

Mel calls, saying, "I'll treat you to a mother/daughter ski day when I visit! Just the two of us!"

Did I hear her correctly? I cry, "Sounds great!"

On Mom's birthday in September I send a card, adding our address and phone number. It hurts that she's making no attempt to contact me.

Oh Abba, I want to trust you with my life, every nook and cranny. Every shelf that needs dusting. Every cobweb needing to be removed. Every dark closet requiring your light. May I be yielded every moment in every way to you. I hear, "*I know your heart, Child. It seeks, it cries after me and I am pleased.*" Oh, that brings me such joy, Abba! I want to please you.

In February, after I enjoy speaking for two women's retreats, Ray flies to Boston and I to Vermont where Anne, Dave, and their two sons now live. We're going to *ski*. My neurologist isn't too keen about it, and Ray's a little scared but backing me. As I ride the lift I'm almost as nervous as my first time skiing with Anne and Dave, but it's like getting back on a bike! I praise God aloud as tears of joy freeze on my face. *TU for the thrill of skiing again and fun with my dear friends!*

It's March 1996. Mel calls to say, "My teacher died and I realize I take so many things for granted. Even though we fight a lot, I really do love you a lot. I would feel terrible if anything happened to you."

Tears pour down my face. "I love you, too. We just need to remember we have lots of great history."

She says, "Yeah."

Ray's new shaped skis immediately give him great form at Mammoth, so he enjoys skiing more than ever. When we arrive home it's obvious Lindsey had a party which she adamantly denies. She's lying pathologically and we feel wrung out. *How do I encourage her when it's difficult to find good?*

Ray says, "It's breaking my heart to see Lins living like this," and I agree.

Then one day I catch her in a lie. Ray says to me, "When are you going to learn? You can't try to explain things to Lins. It feels like badgering. She's not like us. There's something *wrong* with her. Something else is going to have to get through to her."

Lord, I don't want this volley of comments between Lins and me to continue. Empower me with your love.

I'm grateful my voice is in better shape than ever, so I'm checking into recording again. Then bronchitis and laryngitis bombard me. Today I feel weakened all over from the hacking cough, and as I look at my computer screen it reads "I love you, Baby." Tears mist my eyes. Mel, visiting on her spring break, brings me lilies—*TU, Lord!*

Before Mother's Day I send Mom a letter thanking her for the gift of voice lessons *and* the gift of life, adding my number in case she wants to call.

In church I cry over the relationship I *want* to have with Melissia and the sadness I feel about Lindsey's choices. After lunch with Ray I open the letter Mel sent:

"Dear Jo, I wanted to write to you and wish you a happy Mother's Day. It's never been easy for me to call you Mom, or wish you a happy Mother's Day because feelings of betrayal always surface. It still is very confusing having two mother figures around for Mother's Day. I get frustrated in knowing whether or not I should hide my letter of thanks to you, fearing it will upset Mom, but I've been thinking about this and have decided that I don't really care if she finds it. You raised me up since third grade, helped me with my homework, braided my hair, gave me birthday parties, cleaned my owies, took me to school, washed my clothes, made me dinner, supported and helped me with my cookie project in 7th grade, stayed up typing reports when I was too tired to finish, sang me bedtime songs and comforted me when I was sick or if I had had a nightmare, but all around you just loved me unconditionally, even when I was taking you for granted every second. It's been hard having two moms, but I see now, that without you I wouldn't be the person I am today. Thank you for raising me up and dealing with more than you probably bargained for. It means so much. I love you.

Happy Mother's Day. Your Daughter, Melissia Franz"

I'm blinded by tears. So is Ray. *TU, Lord—I will frame it and keep it forever!* In the late evening Mel calls and I say, "Oh, thank you for your wonderful letter. I *cried,* and so did your dad." She says warmly, "I love you" twice. I feel like a bird taken out of a cage of condemnation, and I can fly!

My voice has improved to the point Ray can understand me, but I pray, "Now that I have a gravelly voice I want a clear one." Then I open my mouth to speak to Ray and sound like I'm on a respirator—more air leaks through my vocal chords than words and trying to say a sentence exhausts me! Two specialists say my vocal chords are spasmed open due to an MS attack in my brain.

Melissia calls, "I've been asking God, 'Why your voice?' since you've reached so many. Maybe he wants you to rest because of MS. I know you—when you feel okay you want to be out there."

I say, "Years ago I counseled a woman with MS who couldn't speak and I cried, 'Not my voice, Lord!' then I realized everything I have is his. Though I'm scared, I *have* been praising God. Your call means a lot."

Her voice softens, "I wanted to know you're okay. I love you," and I cry.

Solu-medrol doesn't help. Lins says, "It's not fair. You're always so nice to everyone, and you get sick while all the bad people are out there healthy!"

I quote James 1:2–4, saying, "Maybe I need to learn more perseverance."

She sighs, "Haven't you learned *yet?* Are you a slow learner?" We laugh, but I journal:

> What do you want me to learn? I know I'm to persevere joyfully. I fear losing my voice forever. Not being able to sing and tell of your love. Having my husband struggle to hear me. But you *are* in control. You can use *anything* for your glory. *Do it Lord, I trust you.*

A few days later my friend Barbara drives me to UCLA to see a specialist who examines my vocal chords, then says, "I doubt you will ever sing again."

And he walks out the door.

Chapter 23

Voiceless yet Usable, Still Seeking Mom While Daughter Strays

Those seven words reverberate, taunting. Tears threaten to flow. I sit alone awaiting tests as silent questions torment me—*Abba, have you taken my voice because I've sinned? Do I have a haughty spirit? Have I plunged into ministry and you're slowing me down* ... Suddenly, I'm soothed by my loving Abba's hug, peace surrounds me. That still small voice says, "*Trust me though you are frightened.*"

After Barbara helps me to her car, I weep in her arms, whispering, "I will still praise God."

She states, "That doctor *isn't* God," and I agree.

Ray calls from out of town, shocked and sad. I say, "It's more important for *you* to hear me than for me to sing," while I feel like a songbird robbed of her melody.

> I *do* want to trust you, Lord, but it's *so hard*. I've always been kind and friendly to those who sound like this—with slurred speech and distortion—now I feel humiliated. Please forgive me for my pride and heal me. I have such praises in my heart to sing.

When I call Ruth she can barely hear me, let alone understand. She bursts into tears. Fighting back sobs, I say, "I'll praise God no matter what."

She cries, "Oh, Jo, you don't just know *about* God, you *know* him."

I beg Ray, "Don't quit trying to communicate—I love that in our relationship." He works to read my lips and fine-tunes his listening. We choose restaurants depending upon their loudness, not ambiance or food, sitting closely.

Ray says, "I admire you for the way you're handling this."

I respond, "It's not that I don't feel discouraged, I just don't feel hopeless. God's in control. He knows what's best."

One thing we *can* do is see a movie, so we're watching *Shadowlands* about C. S. Lewis meeting his soul-mate later in life. We're holding hands when Lewis realizes he actually loves Joy *after* she's been diagnosed with terminal cancer. They share a mere three years of intense love and happiness before her death. After his mother died during his childhood, Lewis boarded up his heart. He could've protected himself from the agony of watching a loved one die by insulating himself from loving Joy. Instead, he shared her suffering on a heart-wrenching level. At the end Lewis' character says, "Twice in that life I've been given the choice. As a boy, and as a man. The boy chose safety. The man chooses suffering. The pain now is part of the happiness. That's the deal."[25] As Ray drives, he reaches for my hand. With tear-filled eyes he says he's glad he chose suffering with me. I struggle to say, "Me, too."

Tears well in my eyes this morning as a sacrifice of praise flows from my pen:

"My Voice"

> not really mine at all
> it's yours to use
> to soar in song
> to whisper in darkness.
> My voice
> your voice
> your tool

to silence for your purpose.
May the silence please you
praise you
bring you glory.
Even as embarrassed
as I feel at times
I remember
I want to let you shine.

Lord, *I want to be whole, with no MS. I ask for total healing.* Since you've used MS to touch many, I'm usually at peace, though fearful when it gets bad. I don't understand, but you've allowed this attack. I praise you. I pray to be content if I remain distorted, though it *is* a strain. You care about who I *am*, not what I *do.* I am to *be* for the praise of your glory (Ephesians 1:12). Use me still—publishing is difficult to "break into," but I don't have to succeed to be of worth.

I send off articles and rejection notices return, saying, "Send something else," so I keep submitting, hoping, praying. At the same time I must cancel bookings which I've hardly *ever* done. I don't know when or if I'll speak again.

Answering the phone is difficult—*if* people understand, they usually ask why I'm depressed or crying. Lins explains to her friends, "Mom's having an MS attack on her vocal chords." One day she says, "The way you're handling this makes me want to draw closer to God than any advice you could give." I tear up in gratitude.

Shopping is the worst. I can casually lean on a counter, smiling at others, but when I open my mouth, countenances change abruptly. People who smiled now stare and quickly look away. Clerks crane their necks to hear me, strain to read my lips, then seem to wonder if I'm "all there."

On our ninth anniversary Ray hands me six red and six white long-stemmed roses. He says, "The red ones are for the *fire* in our marriage, and the white are for the *purity* of our commitment." I sigh with love. *TU, Lord, for Ray.*

When Mel brings friends for a visit during the summer, her frequent coldness freezes the warmth wrought by her Mother's Day letter. Meanwhile, pressure constantly mounts with Lindsey while Ray and I are in the cooker. Especially me, since I'm home with Lins who lies habitually, acts irresponsibly and steals. She resents questions, lashing out with a scorpion-tail-tongue to sting me. She demands to be trusted though she isn't trustworthy. She says, "I don't want to deal with you. You're nothing to me but my father's wife!"

I feel slapped back-handed. When she says she wants nothing to do with *us*, Ray says, "Then move out." We suspect her rage and hatred come from drug abuse, but she refuses to be tested.

I call Mom on her birthday and she sounds angry. I explain my voice strangeness is due to MS. I ask if she received my nieces' graduation cards that were returned and I re-sent to her to deliver, if she received her birthday and Christmas cards and the Mother's Day letter.

She says, "No, I did not." She continues, "Well, thank you for wishing me a happy birthday. I'm sorry to hear about your vocal chord problems, Jo."

It doesn't sound like sorrow.

"Goodbye, Jo."

As she hangs up I say, "Goodbye, I love you," and hear in the distance, "I love you," click.

Later I pray, "Lord, Ray and Ruth think since she decided not to respond to anything, she said she never received things. Only you know. Bless her."

Ray and I decide after much prayer to discuss my contacting Mom with a friend who's a counselor. "Jo," she says, "I think you're in bondage to unjustified guilt."

I sigh, "I've been wondering about that."

She asks, "Are you ready to renounce that bondage?"

I say, "*Yes!*" and pray after her to renounce bondage to guilt in the name of Jesus.

When I get a request to speak for a women's conference eighteen months away I write—"TU for hope I'll speak again!" The voice therapist I'm seeing thinks she can help with exercises, and again I thank God.

Then the local MS Society rep says four thespians want to interview someone who has experienced loss due to MS. Their university's theatre department is preparing the play "Duet for One" about Jacqueline Dupree, a famous cellist whose career ended because of MS, so I invite over the three actors and director.

After talking just minutes about my inability to speak and sing, one asks, "Why aren't you angry or depressed?" Silently, I thank God for ordaining this moment. Although I slur my once clear words, speak in a monotone where my voice used to rise and fall naturally, and whisper with low volume, my answer resounds with clarity and power.

"Because I have a relationship with God's Son, Jesus Christ. He loved me enough to die for me, so I can't help but love him in return. The Bible promises, 'In all things God works for the good of those who love him …' (Romans 8:28). I'm not saying I don't feel sad and grieve my losses, but God has proved himself to me in the past."

During the next two hours *they* continue bringing the conversation back to my faith. Two weeks later at the play I tearfully read the dedication to me in the brochure and one of the actors brings me a rose.

But Lindsey's hatefulness grows like a thistle weed.

I need to trust you *every* moment, Spirit, or I'm no different than someone without Christ! I can be just as hurt, immature and hateful. I need to be willing to apologize constantly. The girls are making their choices, and I cannot make anyone happy. I choose your joy. Biological families have just as many difficulties, Christian or not.

Just before Christmas, Lins admits to lying for years about "*everything*" as well as stealing. She's sorry for the meanness she took out on me, and for being so hateful. Then she admits to using drugs.

"I don't deserve to be forgiven and I can't ask for it."

I reach for her. "I forgive you. But our trust is totally broken, and it will take time and proof to rebuild."

By February nothing has improved, and Ray tells Lins the lies have to stop. I feel as if she's telling the truth, so Ray says, "You need to get real. Lins *lies!* She doesn't live in reality!"

Ray and I plan a ski trip to Mammoth to relax in March. On the lift I lean to whisper in his ear, "I'm so excited to be skiing again!" and my mouth drops wide-open—my voice is clear as the cloudless sky! Ray's eyebrows raise, he grins, and hugs me.

Whenever we stop to rest, I cry, "Can you hear me?" My face is frozen in a smile as I continually praise God aloud.

Wow, you are *Lord!* How can I thank you enough for giving me my, no, *your* voice back? And to think I wrote a week ago—"Whatever, use me as you will." My voice therapist is amazed and she loved my testimony tape—I wouldn't have met her otherwise. I read about discipline in Hebrews 12 and ask what I'm to learn. I know you were glorified as others saw your strength in my weakness and fear. You used this to make me more compassionate. I learned *more* perseverance. And you gave me courage to submit writing.

A letter arrives and I open it tentatively to read my story has been accepted for publication in a book, *God's Vitamin "C" for the Hurting Spirit,* compiled by Kathy Collard Miller & D. Larry Miller! *God, you used quiet time for me to become published!* In a week I hear of *another* acceptance.

Our pastor mentions while preaching about a woman who lost her voice for ten months, and what blessed him was the joy she expressed in the midst of her loss. All of a sudden I realize he's speaking of *me,* and I praise God again.

During the loss of my voice, stress mounted with Lindsey, threatening to harden me like hot, molten lava becomes solid. Ray and I prayed nightly, often through tears when we used tough love to say she had to move out again because of the same behavior.

She admitted once, "I've been bitter at you because I've been jealous of you with Dad. I lied to *you* because I knew you believed me." *She covered lies with lies as if one would cancel out the other!* "The reason I've been so mean is the drugs."

She said she would go into rehab and I committed to help her, but she didn't stay with it. Ray and I celebrated ten years of marriage while we wondered if Lins would make it to twenty-one years of age. Acting out of hope, we kept accepting her apologies, letting our revolving-door-daughter return, praying for change. One day I wrote—"I claim 1 Peter 1:3–5 in this trial with Lins. I can *greatly rejoice,* and when I do, my faith grows. If I remember you know what's happening, I can forgive, if not, I *hate* her lying, for it reminds me of others."

Though we decided I was to cease contacting Mom, I send her a Mother's Day card—but *not* out of guilt, explaining that God stopped the attack and I can now speak, signing it, "Love, Jo." Mel calls on Mother's Day, warming my heart, but Lins doesn't. We're just glad she calls the following day so we know she's *alive.* I affirm her having a job, being in rehab and counseling—but we wonder if it's true.

In August I ask Mel if she'd like to go to Catalina Island. She replies, "Oh, I've never been there before; we're going to have so much fun!" While she's visiting, she actually decides to hear me speak, saying afterwards, "You inspired *me,* and I knew what you were going to say!" I'm just thrilled she even wanted to go.

On the ship Melissia and I watch dolphins frolicking, so we reminisce about the time she and her friend were running along the ocean-side, and seeing dolphins, ripped off their shoes to swim with them!

As we lie on a beach she says, "This is one of those memorable moments—seeing your face when you came out of the water after snorkeling the first time." I know my grin was broad.

She goes on, "This was one of the three best days of my life—when you took Lins and me skiing; when I was in Malibu with Jenny, and today. It's perfect. I've always wanted to go to a beach with palm trees and snorkel and be served food."

I smile. *And to think she remembers the time I took them skiing when I couldn't due to my neck! I sat in the lodge and read.* She says she loves the photo album I make for her later.

Meanwhile, Ray's excited to be offered the North American Sales Manager position with a competitor in Fresno, California, but turns it down due to the hot summers because of the MS. I want him happy and challenged in his work, so I encourage him accept it. He doesn't want to travel more because he "loves to be with me," but we know he will. He says, "You're the best thing that ever happened to me. I'm glad we're going on this adventure."

MS kicks in after we arrive in Fresno in November with electrical sensations down not only the front of my legs but my hips when I lower my head; urinary leakage; a woozy feeling in my head and weakness in my arms. My MRI shows a lesion over the area where the C5 damage occurred. Within three weeks I'm delighted symptoms are abating so Ray and I can ski locally in January.

Melissia, now in the Army, wants to come for Christmas. We enjoy a special Christmas Eve in Yosemite, taking part in the small chapel service, and a good Christmas morning, then Mel pushes me away like before. This time I write asking why she treats me like that. In a couple months she tells Ray she's in counseling to "understand why I treat Jo the way I do."

Then Lindsey asks if she can move back in. I actually cry with fear, but we pray for wisdom. On the way home from the airport Ray tells her we believe she can be responsible, but if he catches her lying or stealing she will be "out."

When I think of your greatness my problems shrink to mere annoying gnats. When I forget they appear as giants waiting to crush me. How I want to see you in all your glory. To remember the power that's mine to soar above my concerns. Your love gives me hope that life can be lived on a higher plain than this, where furrows of worry trip me up and I go flying head first into the muck of self-absorption. Let me walk on the hillsides holding your hand. Run on the tundra with an unobstructed view. Even when I cannot see, let me hold your hand, content to be blind, yet led by you. I hear, *"That's what I want from you, Child, trust."*

The few months Lins lives here I'm kind, even when I realize money is missing, because she looks me in the eye and sweetly says she didn't take it. Today I *know* I'm not wrong about missing cash, and Ray says from out-of-town, "Tell her she has to move." Once again *I* have to be "the bad guy."

After praying through my relationship with Mom, I dial her number in April of 1998. I ask how she is.

"Great."

Does she still walk?

"It keeps me going."

I say, "Would you like to consider re-establishing a relationship with me?"

She answers tearfully, "There's been so much hurt. Jo, I love you dearly. I believe Dad did molest you, but I see no relationship coming forward. I have your address and number if I change my mind." Click.

Ray's on the East Coast. I call Ruth and cry. She says, "Your mom lives in the lie that she's a martyr. Her tears have to do with guilt."

Ray later says tenderly, "I'm sorry. I think she still feels guilty for not protecting you."

> I'm sad. I pray Mom opens herself fully to your truth and is freed! I can't imagine life without the enduring purpose to bring you praise and glory. Without enduring hope—how frightening! Without your Spirit's comfort and guidance. Your unconditional love—TU! I hear, *"Child, bask in my love as you are sitting in the sunshine I am providing today."* Yes, it warms the wrinkles of my soul where I've dried up for want of my mother's love. The wrinkles soften as your love's salve moistens and heals. TU for your healing love.

During the Bible study I teach, I talk about soaring while we wait on God as Isaiah 40:41 says, and read my recent prayer:

> I know your presence, your awesome presence. Your overwhelming love. All else palls in comparison. I sense your smile upon me. Your acceptance pours over me like the balm of Gilead. "Thank you" seems too small a

response to such love. You wrap me in the warm cocoon of love to shield me from the enemy's onslaughts on my character, hopes, and dreams. This love empowers me to scale new heights with you. To risk. To dare to dream. I want to share this love with others, to give them hope because you love them so. I smile in return, a timid smile of wonder at your love. I chuckle with the knowledge—it's true, he really does love me this much, and the timid smile broadens into a grin of pleasure."

While I wait for ministry opportunities, I pray:

It's freeing to know you and be freely known. You won't reject me though my thoughts stray to worries I so want to leave at heaven's doorstep so you can sweep them, scatter them like the dust they are—so trivial in the great scheme of things. I'm soaring with you instead of on autopilot. I love you Lord. I hear, "*Do not fear—I will use you again. Shine for me where you are. Enjoy my presence. Wait on me. I am good. I am love. I have your best interests at heart, Child, I love you.*" TU, Abba.

As if giving it all to God is the answer, I hear *Decision* magazine has accepted an article and a story has been accepted for the book *Bounce Back, Too.* Other articles and stories are accepted over the following months. And calls come in for me to speak. Sadly, I turn down two because of trips planned with Ray to New York City and skiing at Whistler, British Columbia. Ray travels too much for me to miss being with him because of speaking. When he calls he says, "I miss you," and I say, "You'd better!" or I say I miss him ... and we laugh. It's a reminder of how important our relationship is.

Now that I'm singing again, Roene and Larry Lettow, and Ray finance my CD, *For the Praise of His Glory,* recorded partially in the studio of my friend Shawna Bryant's husband, Steve. They sacrifice family time and donate recording costs, and yet again I'm overwhelmed and blessed by the loving generosity of friends and my husband. Years ago I decided I couldn't compete in the marketplace with a distributor expecting a heavy touring schedule. I never know when my voice and body will be strong, so I rely totally on God, selling recordings when I speak.

I can't believe it—my sister just called! We haven't talked since she cut off contact. God "told her" to call for years. She asked about everyone in our family *but* me. I buy a cute card expressing how grateful I am, give her my e-mail address and sign it, "With love, Jo." I send her family a Christmas card as well, but never hear from her again.

Since Mel's counseling she's been calling every so often from the Army. I love our talks, especially because she asks for prayer, then tells me how God answered. During a visit Melissia says she no longer wishes her parents were together. She has no regrets that her life happened as it did—she's the person she is because of it. She doesn't want to think what she'd be if she grew up with her mom or if her dad hadn't married me. *TU, Lord.* Then she says, "I never looked at you as a parental figure, only Dad." After she leaves we discuss how she *did* see me as a mother figure.

Over the months Lins and I have been talking occasionally. I apologized for "over-reacting" to things; I just wanted to be a good parent, but tried too hard. She said she stole and lied and did drugs because she was angry at us, mostly *me*. I asked if she was blaming me for her choices. She said, "No, just telling why I made them."

Now our first grandchild is born two weeks after Lins marries the father and I gaze in wonder as I hold our precious, tiny bundle, Calysta. Over the months that follow Lins calls for a recipe and we chat, growing closer. While they're with us for Calysta's first Christmas, Lins ponders aloud, "I can't understand how a woman could ever leave her child."

Our relationship rebuilds, and when we don't hear for awhile we're concerned. When we discover she's separated I say, "I knew something was wrong."

She says, "You knew 'cause you're Mom."

On Mother's Day Mel calls. "I love you and Dad very much. You were good examples of how to make a marriage work in communication with 'I need' and 'I feel' statements. You probably didn't think I was noticing, but I was."

PTL! And she wrote to Ray in a card how grateful she is that he didn't abandon her. Ray thinks she's admitting her mom *did,* and without that, he says, "She can't become whole."

The MS has weakened my back and neck so much I lie on the floor frequently to adjust them with two tennis balls taped together as a PT taught me, because I feel a pinching pain from the misaligned vertebra. I stretch out spasmed, tight, painful muscles, as well. I awaken often and must do the same things on a sheet covering the carpet. When I go away to speak or travel with Ray my floor-sheet goes along.

While we take a trip to Crater Lake, then down the incredibly unique Oregon coastline, we have little time together. Ray leaves phone messages, "From your not-so-secret-admirer." Inga and Ruben visit, enamored by the huge sequoia trees and Yosemite National Park while Ray bonds even closer to them. By spring of our third year in Fresno, Ray and I tire of his constant travel. When he's offered a position in Portland, Oregon, with the promise of less traveling, he gladly accepts.

Suddenly, I need surgery on an abscess, then an MS exacerbation grabs my central nervous system with each faltering, shaking, grappling step to find the floor, while I push my wheelchair for support. I assure Ray he should attend a dental convention since our small Bible study group commits to bring meals, plus a nurse comes twice a day to clean the wound.

> Oh, dear Abba, I love crawling up in your lap. When life gets tough and peace eludes me, I draw close. When pain frays my nerves and tears sting my eyes, your arms reach out to place me where no abuse is found, only your tender touch. You wipe my tears, stroke my hair, and tell me you love me. I release all the hurt and fear and relax. My heart beats slower. TU, Daddy. I hear, *"Child, I love you."* I know you do!

Numerous men ask Ray about his upcoming job change, and his answer impacts them more than Ray could've imagined. One said, "It's great you're putting your wife ahead of your career," and Ray tells me he said, "She's worth it! She's a jewel!"

I'm still recovering from the several-week-long MS attack when we move to Southwest Washington, just north of Portland.

After flying to California for several speaking engagements, I receive a note from a young woman whose aunt brought her to hear me, but she planned on checking into a hotel to kill herself afterwards. She wanted to run down the aisle after I spoke to hug me through tears and tell me, "Now I don't have to die!" Tearful joy humbles me.

By December my sleep pattern has been so disrupted by frog-leg-spasm-pain that I live in a fog. I begin seeing a PT, an OT, and a rehab director. Armed with a cervical MRI and x-rays, he explains that if I fall I could easily be rendered a quadriplegic, cautioning me against skiing.

Tears fill my eyes, and he looks away when I say, "This is hard. I love to ski. I feel graceful and free and I praise God." But I tell him I'm not stupid. I *know* how it feels to *not* feel anything from the neck down when I had the xylocaine drug reaction and when I tumbled down the stairs.

In the car I cry out, "You know I love to ski, Lord. I don't want to stop, but you've given me years of wonderful memories."

> I know instinctively this is right, but *why* take it away when I praise you? When I witness to others of your strength and give you glory? I don't understand. Where is the greater praise opportunity? When I ski, or say it's a lost love for which I praise you anyway? I seek *your* wisdom, your heart, your mind. I hear that soft voice, "*Protect yourself and I will use you, Child. Trust me.*" I *will* praise you. Use my loss for your glory.

Though I try one prescription after another over months, spasms jolt me awake like earthquakes. The attack after surgery last year left me with such ataxic walking, that I depend upon my cool-aids more than ever. I've developed arthritis in my wrists, fingers, and especially my thumbs from years of trying to stay mobile with crutches. The doctor thinks I'll need thumb joint replacements if I continue using crutches, and I might not regain strength in my hands and arms after the immobilization following surgery. A PT explained once, that with MS, after a week's lack of movement one begins losing musculature. That's why I've tried to exercise five to six days a week. For several years I've had chronic tendonitis in my elbows, with shoulder pain as well. Now I'm experiencing numbness in toes, fingers, and around my mouth with my head buzzing constantly. *TU, God, I get around as well as I do!*

My neurologist says, "You're doing better than you should be!"

I say, "I believe my faith in God and exercise has something to do with that."

I know it's your grace and my listening to you.

You love me so much! Your thoughts of me (Psalm 139) swirl around like a deliciously cool stream bubbling delightfully in which I sit. How I love your love! The Spirit's voice says, "*Child, let my love cover you. Lap it up. Delight in it. Never fear when I am with you.*"

I'm so tired of being tired from lack of sleep and drug-grogginess, and I grieve the loss of skiing, but that's nothing compared to how Inga and Ruben feel about his cancer. Our hearts go out to them on the other side of the world so we call often. Meanwhile, Mel tracked down Ray's older daughter, Mandy, and she's written him. We're elated!

Almost a week after I'm overwhelmed with happy Mother's Day calls from *both* Mel and Lins, I pray, "I'm exhausted. I'm begging you to show me any emotional or spiritual problem causing me to wake up in pain."

I hear, "*Child, it is not you. I am allowing MS for a greater purpose.*"

I respond, "You know how I've tried to share my witness with everyone, but I fear it's faltering due to sleep deprivation and pain-induced depression," but I sense, "*Child, I can work in that weakness.*"

I lie awake with my legs jerking like a caffeinated frog. Ray prayed for me to get a good night's sleep, now he snores softly as I pray, "You know what I need. I'm looking forward to what you'll do." Then the Spirit lays on my mind Isaiah 40:31—"Those who hope in the Lord will renew their strength. They will soar on wings like eagles ..."

Suddenly, it's as if I'm looking down from the wings of an eagle on which I sit! I soar over Longs Peak which I climbed. We swoop down, then soar over the trail I hiked crossing the Continental Divide, then fly all over

Rocky Mountain National Park I've explored, backpacking. We dive into valleys and catch thermals up high. Then we soar over Winter Park where I look down on disabled skiers among able-bodied ones. I'm singing "The Power of Your Love"[26] about flying like eagles and I don't want our flight to end! It seems I ease down onto the bed and lie here basking in God's love while the rest of the night my legs hop and I get little sleep. In the morning I barely stay awake in church, lie down as soon as we get home, go to my office, sit in my rocker, and journal:

> Oh, Abba, TU for the *wonderful* time. When I told Ray, he said he wishes he could soar on an eagle! The significance of where you took me is so powerful—over trails I can no longer hike and ski runs—lost loves. For months I've grieved the loss of skiing. What do you want me to learn? I hear, *"As you soar with me, waiting for heaven, all your losses mean nothing in comparison."* I knew that! TU for this reminder—*nothing* compares to soaring in relationship with you! Is this what you want me to be sharing? That sweet voice speaks to my heart, *"Yes, Child. There will be losses and grief, but I am always with you."*

Chapter 24

Learning to Soar Unafraid

Pain accompanies me daily now, but when I'm worn down, I cry out to God and his loving arms wrap around me so I soar above pain and fatigue. Ever since the night on eagle's wings I haven't had a frog-leg spasm! I still wake with muscle tightness in my legs and groin, which I stretch out before adjusting my back, but I don't jerk awake. I'm getting slightly better sleep and feel overflowing with gratitude.

On my birthday Inga calls to say Ruben went home to Jesus. We comfort each other through tears. Ray and I phone every month to exhort her to live for Christ—she can't give up, while we must deal with a unique challenge.

Ray faces a work crisis for the *first* time. As we pray fervently, we also praise God because of who he is—sovereign Lord of all. The company asks us to move to Salt Lake City for a year, so I say, "Well, maybe God has people for us to meet there just like all the other places we've lived."

Ray says teary-eyed, "I know I just want what God wants." He pauses, then continues, "This has changed me. It's taken this for me to see I didn't want *whatever* God wanted before. I wasn't trusting. Now I want to be in God's will more than anything."

I tear up, "I've been praying that for you for *years.*"

"It's taken me a long time. I've sensed God's love more profoundly than ever before because of being vulnerable with him." I'm thrilled for Ray.

In January I have the privilege of being the keynote speaker for nearly six hundred women at the Northern California Baptist Conference, having presented a workshop two years earlier while we lived in Fresno. A woman with tear-soaked-face grabs me after I speak, saying, "Now I don't want to kill myself!" The prayer room fills with women seeking to know Christ more intimately, and I'm overwhelmed to be God's instrument.

While in Utah we travel to Sweden to see Inga. Her son, Anders, tells us later he's grateful our visit changed her attitude about life. All we do is love her and respond to her abundant love, but she entertains for the first time in nearly two years to invite my dear friends to meet Ray. He's welcomed with loving arms and hearts, and Inga's sense of purpose to help others is renewed. Ray and I love being in Sweden together, and I'm excited to share in Kyrka vid Brommaplan's church service, which I've done over the years. I can't walk while sight-seeing as I did my last trip, but Ray pushes me lovingly in a borrowed wheelchair. On buses he puts *his* "baby" in the baby stroller area.

The year flies by as we behold changing colors of aspen leaves in the mountains; revel in snowfall, and a hillside of mountain goats. But on Christmas day Melissia calls with news she says will disappoint us—because we taught both daughters what God desires in order to *bless* us. We're to become grandparents again, and Mel isn't married.

I tell Melissia we'll love her child and look forward to his or her coming.

Over the following months Mel tries to work it out with her baby's father, but ultimately feels it best they don't marry. She leaves the Army when she receives a great job offer due to the military training she excelled in.

Two days before we're to leave Utah for Washington, our friend Kay prays with me over the phone to become a Christian, leaving the LDS faith for a new life with Jesus. Over the preceding months both Ray and I shared our faith with Kay. *She* was the reason we were sent to Utah, and we're overjoyed to have been used in her life, as well as her husband's.

In June I receive a touching birthday card from Mom. I'm shocked, like I was six months ago with the first Christmas card I'd received in fourteen years (though I always sent them). She wrote, "Sorry you never make it back," and we couldn't understand *why* she would write something so naïve unless she was losing touch with reality. Flood gates had opened just before receiving her card. I wrote that Thanksgiving:

> I weep so deeply sobs become choked notes emitting from the top of my vocal chords. You love me, but my birth-family doesn't. When my family shut off contact, I lost precious relationships with nieces and nephews. I've always wondered what they told the children. I didn't know this scar hadn't healed. Do they feel the void of *my* absence? I can't see to write. I hear you say, "*I provide people like Ray with skin on to love you, but I meet your deepest needs.*" TU, Abba.

I ponder calling Mom when we go to Colorado to see Melissia's son after his birth in August. How fascinating Mom wrote just when I've decided to put all my energy into my memoir—years ago I tried, but wasn't ready. Now I hear, "*Soar unafraid as you write. Be vulnerable and soar unafraid!*"

Mandy visits in August, seeing her dad for the first time in nearly twenty years. As are Lindsey and Melissia, Mandy's beautiful, and at six feet tall with Ray's dark hair and the same eyes, she looks most like him of the three. When Ray asks her forgiveness for not being in her life more when she was younger, she hugs him, saying, "You're forgiven, Dad. I love you."

Mandy doesn't blame him for the past sixteen years—that was *her* choice due to her lifestyle. Their tearful talks over the past few months led up to this.

I adopt Mandy, and when she says, laughing, "You don't let anything get past each other! You don't always agree but you work it out," I thank God. While leaning against the cool wall talking with Mandy, I notice a strange numbness in my left knee and thigh, but don't call my doctor since he saves steroids for worse attacks. I ignore it.

In early September Ray and I are talking with friends when my left knee collapses and I can't straighten it. I felt fatigued, but I'm startled by Ray's need to put his arm around me and mine him as he half-drags me to the car. In the morning I can't walk! Immediately, I call my neurologist who sees me that afternoon.

He says, "The numbness was probably the precursor. I think there's a large lesion in your spinal cord."

I begin five days of out-patient IV-Solu-medrol. When I send a quick e-mail to my Praying Friends I write—"I'm the weakest I've been in nine years—since my stair-dive and subsequent MS attacks—but Ray and I wait on tiptoe to see what God is going to do next because He *is* in control."

The following Monday I'm *weaker*. Ray buys a porta-potty, then after three *more* infusions I feel a tiny bit of strength returning. I'm still so limp I lean my neck against a pillow since I can't hold my head up for long. The daily nerve fiber pain circling my torso now feels like I've burned myself. Muscle spasms constantly grab my back and neck, though I praise God through tears. My next e-mail says:

"This morning as we worshipped at home, I closed my eyes and shakily sang through weakened vocal chords a song about Jesus holding healing in his hands.[27] I saw what appeared to be Jesus reach towards me. I weakly journaled—'TU Jesus, for your love reaching out to me with your touch of healing,' and I heard, '*Child, I am your healing.*' God—knowing him—is my healing. Not mere physical healing. Emotional, spiritual, *whole* healing is found in him. He is the *I am* for life. No matter what happens to us Jesus is the *I am* that we need. And I rest in him with joy and peace."

Ray tenderly washes and dries my hair. He adds doing everything else to the grocery shopping, which he's done for years. Then he rents a scooter since I still can't walk, and he must go out-of-town weekly. Our precious friends—Bible study group, church, and others—bring meals, and our neighbor has a key if I need her. On his way home Ray calls and sings the theme line from the song "Working My Way Back to You,"[28] saying he has that same burning love for me. Tears moisten my eyes.

But even when I'm alone I don't feel blue. It's as if God reaches in and massages my heart with his hand of love. Outside our windows, fall splendor amazes me with a golden-rod leaf fluttering down on a waft like a lone yellow snowflake. I notice for the first time a tree trunk with a graceful curve, and I'm reminded God's beauty is found not through perfection—straight trunks—but through his strength in imperfect vessels, like me. Blue jays sing and caw to welcome me each morning with God's grace. I hear, *"My child, my creation is a gift for you to enjoy. I am pleased with your praise. Enjoy my gift today and always."*

Now I seem to wear a leaded hula-skirt when I walk tentatively, pushing the wheelchair. At least I'm walking! Five weeks after the attack hit, my PT sadly notes how weak I am, but I respond, "I *will* work to regain strength." Within a week my doctor fears I'm in yet another MS attack. I deplore the Solu-medrol that feels like an angry bee dwells in me. Ray's in San Francisco, teasing, "Can't you time these attacks better?" He calls to say, "You're riding on the cable car with me, baby!" I smile because he's thinking of me "always."

We feel saddest when we go to church while I'm in my wheelchair, and friends we usually chat with stand away, as if we're contagious, even pastors. One of the guys in our small group touches Ray's heart when he asks, "How are *you* holding up?" Later, Ray tells the group how scared he was. "I didn't know if my wife would ever walk again. Our whole lifestyle could be changing." *We've been here before, Lord, thank you once again.*

As the flare-up finally lets up, I make myself walk, pushing the wheelchair a short distance every thirty minutes, until I cry tears of exhaustion. I exercise a little more, then see my PT.

Lisa cries, "Jo, your muscles remember what to do because you've trained them by faithful exercise!"

God, you put the desire in me and I listen. I praise you!

I realize during these months I've been privileged to humbly live in

God's glory—in his presence—more than ever. How can I not thank him for these months of the "MS siege," as a friend calls it?

> Ray thinks I have awe about your love because of my past. Or is it because I've nurtured my love and awe for you, Abba? I hear, "*It is our relationship, my child. You do not take it for granted. That is why you hear my voice and know my love.*" Your love empowers me to have peace in the midst of storms. To rejoice in who you are rather than give in to fear. To soar unafraid and not become bitter. You are my life.

Before Thanksgiving I call Mom to thank her for the cards and she's *nice!* She repeats herself, though, and seems to lose track conversing. I sense God urging me to visit, but can't until I'm stronger. Then our family arrives and Ray and I rejoice to have *all* of us together, including Mandy. Our prayers of years have finally been answered.

In April Ray and I fly to California, and like last time, we spend delightful hours with Lindsey, granddaughter Calysta, and Lins' boyfriend, Jesse. We see such positive changes in Lins we're not sure how to react, except with love and joy. She and I love chatting long-distance.

As we await our return flight, a tall lean man comes over, introducing himself as Hank, someone Ray knows in the dental industry.

Hank says, "I want to tell you, I don't know *any* man who is more in love with his wife than Ray, or more proud of her."

I smile in awe and say, "Thank you. Ray's a blessing to me, too," as I reach for Ray's hand. I tell him on the plane how loved I feel that he must be wearing his feelings about me on his sleeve for other men to see.

Ray and I are eating lunch, having worked in our respective home offices, which we enjoy, when I say, "I sense God telling me to see Mom. You've been through it all with me. I don't want to go alone."

"I have no desire to be in her presence," he states. "Are you going to try to make me feel guilty about this?"

"No. I just hope it's not because of bitterness because that will affect your relationship with the Lord." We leave the table and I pray.

In about twenty minutes Ray walks in, saying, "I checked flights and hotel cost. I'll be glad to go with you to your mom's."

I get up to kiss and hug him as he holds me tightly. I say, "You're a great guy," tears choking my voice, and he responds, "Sometimes." I laugh, "Well, you work your way there. Who knows but God why I feel led to go."

After we set the date, I ask my Praying Friends to pray for God's will in the visit, and for me as I read through my journal entries of the memories before we go. I want to be certain I'm totally healed, with no unresolved issues or bitterness that could be triggered in Mom's presence. At 9:00 p.m. the night before we fly I finish. Ray and I tear-up when I read him parts about his support during what I went through to become whole, and *his* amazing healing along with me.

Ray leaves me at the airport terminal while he rents a car, then picks me up in a canary-yellow Mustang convertible! Our first stop is to visit Melissia and active little Aiden, whose huge blue eyes twinkle—and what a joyful time it is. Mel had written expressing her hurt and anger about our parenting only months before. We sincerely apologized for what we felt responsible, and though that didn't completely satisfy her, we're grateful she's loving.

During the night I wake frequently with nightmares, praising God as I remind myself I've put on his armor (Ephesians 6:13–17)—I'm in the midst of spiritual warfare. Memories flood over me as we drive to Mom's.

Ray supports my left arm with his right, like he does now that my left thumb is so arthritic, and I ring the doorbell. Mom appears, wrinkled, with gray hair, and I say, "Mom, it's Jo."

She looks confused, saying, "I think I recognize you."

Then she asks, "What did you do to your hair?"

I laugh inside because I'd just told my hairdresser Mom's never liked my hair unless it's short, and she'll probably comment.

While Ray sits with her, I head to the bathroom where I relive a memory and tell myself *don't think about it—no, it's alright—it can't hurt me.* I suggest we sit outside where I show her photos of our family and house. As we talk about the family I no longer know, she repeats sentences. *She must have dementia.* I ask about Dad's death and she's lucid, saying her typical, "I don't think about those things. I just put them out of my mind." I ask about things that happened years before I left home and she's clear. I think I could bring up what divided us and she would remember, but feel no need.

When we come inside to take Mom to lunch, my sister unexpectedly appears. Rhonda's friendly and we hug, but she's taking Mom to a hair appointment, and I can't fathom why it can't be rescheduled.

Rhonda says, "She's already forgotten once. She has Alzheimer's. Her sister died of it recently."

I complement Rhonda about being supportive to Mom, then we get to Rhonda's car. Confusion covers Mom's face, so I say, "I'm sorry you have a hair appointment and we can't take you to lunch." Ray and I both hug her. Then I hug my sister and tell them both, "I love you," and say good-bye.

As we drive away we both feel sad about Mom's turmoil, then Ray says, "She has no power over you."

I smile because *he's right!* I can *soar* without guilt about bringing up the truth! We drive to Idaho Springs, exclaiming when we spot mountain sheep rams alongside the highway butting heads.

Later, I call Mom, saying, "It was good to see you."

"It was great to see you! I want you to know I'm proud as a peacock about you."

"Thank you, Mom."

"You tell Ray I think you two are doing great."

I tell her if we have time we'll come by again and I love her.

Over dinner with Peg and Hal we discuss seeing Mom and Rhonda. They agree there was closure and a sort of blessing given. Hal says, "Every time I pick up to read *The Survivor Personality*[29] I think of *you*," and he hugs me.

They, as well as Ruth and Ken, suggest we don't visit Mom again. What fun to see our good friends! And driving through the mountains we love in the convertible, seeing a herd of elk and mountain goats along with a moose and her calf, absolutely thrills us.

MS relapses again in August, and after IV-Solu-medrol in the clinic, where I love to share my faith, I hear from my neurologist the same thing I was told years ago, that I'm probably going into Secondary-Progressive MS. I've lost at least seven months over these past eighteen to MS, halting my writing. Then it took time before I could build up strength to sit at the computer (at best a few hours interrupted by a nap). I even tried a voice-activated program, but found it constraining to my creativity. And I needed to rebuild my vocal chord strength so I can continue speaking and singing. I *know* I'm not as strong as before, even as I continue injecting Betaseron. My doctor encourages me to additionally take a chemo called Novantrone to halt MS progression. I consent and end up sick and weak for a month with a virus I can't shake due to my low white blood cell count. Three months later, after the second treatment, I'm ill with what might be pneumonia. Pin-prick pain continues around my eyes as well as stabbing pains in my eyeballs along with overall fatigue—at least I can see, but I'm not accomplishing much.

> I want to freefall from a high bridge into your arms. I just want to trust you that much! Oh Abba, help me in my unbelief that tells me I'm not useable when I *know* you use me if I'm yielded. I hear, *"My child, I am using you where you are. Sit at the mountain of my love for you. It is greater than you can see past. You cannot fathom my love for you. Feast on it. Soar unafraid while you wait!"*

When my purple power wheelchair is delivered, I ask Ray to take pictures of me in it as I smile joyfully. I'm finally *glad* to have this, having grieved the need for it to even get mail from our box only a house away. I just can't walk that far using my cool-aids without pain and wearing out my thumb joints. I'm learning to soar unafraid of further weakness as I use the chair because God knows my condition. When I'm finally over the infection, I gradually exercise on a large ball and become a little stronger, able to write for longer periods, though still only a few hours a day, and I can walk short distances using my crutches, though I do better with help supporting my left arm and hand due to arthritis.

My most recent MRIs show no new activity with incredibly light density-lesions, a huge improvement from before, and we're delighted! My neurologist has no explanation since I took chemo eighteen months ago. I say, "Well, God did it!" and for once, he agrees, "Yes—God!"

As I write, I trust God to provide all I need, just as I do speaking and singing, soaring unafraid, letting him use me as he chooses. Like Rae Reed, director of the NCBC Women's Ministries, wrote, "In spite of your health challenges, you minister with an energy and determination that are a testimony of God's faithfulness to you." It is *God's* strength, not mine. I love to write my Praying Friends about how God worked through their prayers! As friends continue to drive me to engagements, or assist me when I fly, I'm constantly grateful. After several years since my soaring on eagles wings experience, I *still* don't have any knee-jerk spasm frog-leg jumps—PTL!

During our next visit with Lins, now with a darling new curly, red-headed daughter, Maycn, Lins and I talk about *our* family. She says, "I've watched a lot of counseling programs and our family did so many things wrong. Dad should've never put you in an authoritative role, it created anger ..."

Later, I tell Ray and he says, "If I had it to do all over again, I'd do the same thing."

In the morning Lindsey says, "I've been thinking about it, and you had no choice but to discipline us 'cause Dad traveled. Like you said, you were just trying to establish a family like we all wanted. They know a lot more about step-families now than they did back then."

I'm grateful for her trying to understand and give us grace. I'm also touched because she's now sorrowful over her past behavior that wreaked such havoc in our lives.

I sit on my stool before the appropriately-painted mural of *The Velveteen Rabbit* story, with my own green velveteen rabbit Lins sewed for me in high school nearby. I tell the audience of mothers and daughters how our family came to be, and some of the fun, loving times when my fur was rubbed off. Then I share how Melissia told me she wanted to call me "Jo."

I say, "I'd like to tell you I handled it like Christ would have wanted me to. I did not. Though I prayed, I felt my 'velveteen mom' status being stripped, and I reacted wrongly. When Melissia moved to her mother's, I felt totally responsible. Then I received this letter," and I read the Mother's Day letter from Mel.

A woman in the front announces, "You should frame that!" and I say the original *is* framed.

I go on, "Families are messy." Around the room, women nod. "No matter how hard we try, they don't always turn out like we want. Without Christ we can't be the parents we should be, and even then we sometimes fail. I'm so glad God forgives. Without him I would be nothing." Then I end by singing, "In Christ Alone."

In a couple months I write Melissia to ask her forgiveness with deep and sincere sorrow for not handling it like Christ—and I—wanted, when she called me "Jo." Years ago I had such trouble forgiving myself. Now I can rest—knowing it was wrong, though provoked by my past hurts and family rejection—because Melissia forgives me. I ask God to use it together for our good somehow, because I *know* he can use even our mistakes.

I've made so many. I was too needy myself as a parent, but I now soar without condemnation because when I admit my sin, I *know* I am forgiven. "Therefore, there is now no condemnation for those who are in Christ Jesus" (Romans 8:1). I so want to grant that to others. I call Mom every so often to chat and so far she still knows me.

In our prayers, Ray and I are learning to soar unafraid of the future as we trust Philippians 4:6–7—"Do not be anxious about anything, but in everything, by prayer and petition, *with thanksgiving,* present your requests to God. And the peace of God, which transcends all understanding, will guard your hearts and your minds in Christ Jesus" (italics mine). We're all excitedly looking forward to Lindsey and Jesse's upcoming wedding, and Melissia and Aiden are visiting churches—years of prayers are being answered—not in our time—in God's.

As I gave chapters of this memoir to Ray, tears filled his eyes, and he said he was so sorry he had hurt me *and* the girls when they moved away, not realizing the depth of their love for me. He'd never let *any* of the few women he dated close to them until me, and he says he couldn't have protected them—because though he feared a relationship so much he now knows he would've run until God worked on him—Ray believed from the first date that I was meant for him. And that meant the girls had to know me. Ray would never have married anyone who didn't love his daughters, or they her. He was also shocked to realize how messed up he was—he'd forgotten during these past years of profound growth.

We continue to hold each other accountable, reminding each other often how glad we are to have one another by nurturing our love. After twenty years of marriage we can hardly believe how blessed we are. We soar unafraid as we continue to learn how to love each other fully in the love of God.

I want to live in your grace this day. I want to bring a smile to your face and I sense it. My heart beats with the joy of knowing you. Of being *your* child—loved, forgiven, redeemed, and one day blessed with a home in heaven, forever, with you. There are days when I long for that place of perfect rest, perfect hope, perfect fellowship with you. Until then I persevere with your strength. Your hope for the future. Your peace for today. Your love wrapping around my heart, squeezing life, your perfect, transcending life, into it so I can soar unafraid. Thank you, my Lord, my Abba, my friend, and I hear, *"You are welcome, Child."*

Acknowledgements

This has been in the birthing stage for some time. My memoir is a book of truth as I remember it, most of which comes from journal entries. Though I have changed a few names, descriptions, and places, this does not detract from its truthfulness.

Thanks to all of you who have heard me speak, then asked that I write my story. I hope you find it's been worth the wait—there was so much more to tell after the first request twenty-three years ago.

To my faithful editors, Jessica Shaver Renshaw and Cindy Rivans, thanks for hanging in month after month as I sent chapters; giving your critical input, emotional responses, and encouragement.

To additional readers: Erin Campbell, Katie Croskrey, Lynda Libby, Phil Miller, Gary Thomas, Lisa Thomas, and Sandra Wilson, your insights and hope have been invaluable.

And Ruth Peters, dear friend, you've read and edited parts of this through the years, always pushing me forward with assurance that it can reach and touch the hearts of many—thank you.

Special thanks to Barbara and John Cosgrove, Ray Franz, Kay and Doug Jackman, and Roene and Larry Lettow. Your belief in this book gave it wings to soar.

Friends have enriched my life beyond dreams. While I've written about a few, there's no way I could name you all. My included song is dedicated to each and every one of you, named and unnamed—how can I thank you enough for being my wheels, supporting and visiting me when I've been laid up, bringing meals, making ministry possible, *literally* lifting and carrying me so I could experience an amazing life on a level many with disabilities never do. You are precious in God's sight and mine.

Soar Unafraid would not have been written without my amazing Praying Friends battling for me—God knows who you are and your faithful hearts of intercession. Bless you.

I would also like to thank the many doctors, nurses, physical and occupational therapists I've been blessed to have been treated by—you are unsung heroes in my book.

I've been touched emotionally and spiritually by many "counselors." Though I couldn't name each of you, know that your compassionate listening and discernment have been used to hone me into the person I am today, and I'm so grateful.

I've enjoyed interacting with each of the Tate staff who helped make this book reality—Ryan Tate, Rita Tate, Dave Dolphin, Jennifer Bass, my encouraging editor who didn't want readers to "miss anything," Sarah Leis, who took our cover ideas then transformed them beautifully, and Jennifer Redden, whose layout enhances the reading experience, thanks for partnering with me.

I especially want to thank my husband, Ray, who lights every day with laughter and love, who took the risk of marrying me with MS and never looked back, sharing burdens and joys immeasurable. He and our cat, Jaz, have put up with a lot as I've worked on this manuscript.

Thank you, also, Ray, for giving me the gift of being a stepmother to our wonderful daughters, Lindsey and Melissia. Through it all, I never doubted it was a privilege. I love you.

And last, but foremost, I thank my God, my one and only loving Daddy, who gives me overflowing love every day of life that I wouldn't even be experiencing without you.

Notes

Chapter 1

1   "Both Sides Now," copyright © 1967 (Renewed) Crazy Crow Music. Words and music by Joni Mitchel.

2   Joni Eareckson Tada & Joe Musser, copyright © 1976, 1996, 2001 *Joni* (Grand Rapids: Zondervan, 2001).

Chapter 2

3   Joni Eareckson & Steve Estes, copyright © *A Step Further* (Grand Rapids: Zondervan Publishing House, 1978).

4   "But You *LOOK* So Good," National Multiple Sclerosis Society Facts & Issues, Department of Medical and Community Services, Number 1.

5   "It Is Well with My Soul," copyright © 1873 Words by Horatio G. Spafford and copyright © 1876 Music by Philip P. Bliss.

Chapter 3

6   "And Then Come the Friends," copyright © 1983, Words and Music by Jo, Recording copyright © 1988 by Jo Franz.

7   William Backus & Marie Chapian, copyright © *Telling Yourself The Truth* (Minneapolis: Bethany House, 1985).

8   Dr. James C. Dobson, copyright © *Love Must Be Tough* (Dallas: Word, Incorporated, 1983).

9   "The Journey," copyright © 1977 Triune Music, Inc. Words by Ragan Courtney and Music by Cynthia Clawson, ASCAP.

10   Jim Smoke, copyright © *Suddenly Single* (Grand Rapids: F. H. Revell Co., 1982).

Chapter 8

11   Taylor-Johnson Temperament Analysis® measures personality traits.

Chapter 9

12   "You've Brought Me Through Heartache … to Soaring on Broken Wings," copyright © 1986 Words and Music by Jo. Recording copyright © 1988 by Jo Franz.

13   "He Knows," copyright © 1986 Words and Music by Jo. Recording copyright © 1988 by Jo Franz.

Chapter 10

14   Elisabeth Kubler-Ross, M.D., *On Death and Dying*, copyright © 1967 by Elisabeth Kubler-Ross, M.D. (New York: Touchstone, 1997).

Chapter 12

15   David Augsburger, *Caring Enough to Confront* (copyright © 1973 under the title *The Love Fight* by Herald Press, Scottdale, PA; Ventura: Regal Books, 1983).

Chapter 14

16   Judith S. Seixas & Geraldine Youcha, copyright © *Children of Alcoholism/ A Survivor's Manual* (New York: Crown Publishers, Inc. 1985).

Chapter 15

17   John Powell, *Why Am I Afraid to Love?* (Niles: Argus, 1967, Revised 1972)

Chapter 16

18   "Household of Faith," Words and Music by Brent Lamb and John Rosasco, copyright © 1983 StraightWay Music.

19   David A. Seamands, copyright © *Healing of Memories* (Wheaton: Victor Books, Second printing, 1985).

20   *Caring Enough to Confront.*

21   Dr. David Stoop & Dr. James Masteller, copyright © *Forgiving Our Parents Forgiving Ourselves* (Ann Arbor, MI: Servant Publications, 1991). Lewis B. Smedes, copyright © *Forgive and Forget, Healing the Hurts We Don't Deserve* (San Francisco: Harper & Row, 1984).

Chapter 18

22   "My Heart Wants to Cry Out, Lord!" copyright © 1985, 1986 Words and Music by Jo, Recording copyright © 1988 by Jo Franz.

23   Margery Williams, *The Velveteen Rabbit* (NY: Doubleday & Company, Inc., 1922).

24   Marilyn Van Derbur, "The Darkest Secret," People Weekly, June 10, 1991: 88–94.

Chapter 23

25   *Shadowlands*, DVD, director Richard Attenborough, editor Lesley Walker, Sony Pictures, Inc., 1993.

26   "Power of Your Love," copyright © 1992 Word Music (a div. of WORD, Inc.) ASCAP, by Geoff Bullock.

Chapter 24

27   "It is You," copyright © 1999 Darlene Zschech/Hillsong Publishing, Australia.

28   "Working My Way Back to You," copyright © 1966 Sandy Linzer & Denny Randell.

29   Al Siebert, Ph.D., copyright © 1993, 1994, *The Survivor Personality* (New York: A Perigee Book published by The Berkley Publishing Group, 1996).